Seminar Participants

Paul Dyment, MD
Chief of Pediatrics
Department of Pediatrics
Maine Medical Center
Portland, Maine

James Farmer, PhD
Associate Professor of Continuing
    Education
College of Education
University of Illinois
Champaign, Illinois

Carlos Garcia-Moral, MD
Clinical Professor
Department of Orthopaedics and
    Rehabilitation
University of Oklahoma
Health Sciences Center
Oklahoma City, Oklahoma

James Garrick, MD
Director
Center for Sports Medicine
St. Francis Memorial Hospital
San Francisco, California

William Grana, MD
Clinical Professor
Department of Orthopaedic Surgery and
    Rehabilitation
University of Oklahoma College of
    Medicine
Oklahoma City, Oklahoma

Richard Gross, MD
Associate Professor and Vice Chairman
Department of Orthopaedics
Medical University of South Carolina
Charleston, South Carolina

William Herndon, MD
Associate Professor
Department of Orthopaedics
Oklahoma Children's Hospital
Oklahoma City, Oklahoma

Tony Herring, MD
Texas Scottish Rite Hospital
Dallas, Texas

Letha Hunter-Griffin, MD, PhD
Orthopaedic Surgeon
Atlanta, Georgia

Frank Kulling, MD
Assistant Professor, HPELS
Oklahoma State University
Stillwater, Oklahoma

John Lombardo, MD
Medical Director
Section of Sport Medicine
Department of Orthopaedic Surgery
The Cleveland Clinic Foundation
Cleveland, Ohio

John Meyers, MD
Orthopaedic Surgeon
Richmond, Virginia

Lyle Micheli, MD
Director
Division of Sports Medicine
The Children's Hospital
Boston, Massachusetts

Michael Nelson, MD
Associate Clinical Professor of Pediatrics
University of New Mexico
Albuquerque, New Mexico

Bruce Ogilvie, PhD
Professor Emeritus
Psychology Department
San Jose State University
Los Gatos, California

Peter Pizzutillo, MD
Director, Pediatric Orthopaedic Surgery
Associate Professor of Orthopaedic Surgery
    and Pediatrics
Thomas Jefferson University
Philadelphia, Pennsylvania

Don Porter, Executive Director
Amateur Softball Association
Oklahoma City, Oklahoma

Ronald Ratliff, PhD
Associate Professor
University of Oklahoma
Norman, Oklahoma

Brian Sharkey, PhD
Dean, College of Human Performance
University of Northern Colorado
Greeley, Colorado

Carl Stanitski, MD
Clinical Associate Professor
Department of Orthopaedics
University of Pittsburgh
Pittsburgh, Pennsylvania

J. Andy Sullivan, MD
Professor, Chief
Pediatric Orthopaedic Surgery
University of Oklahoma Health Sciences
  Center
Oklahoma City, Oklahoma

Dee Tipton, MPH, PT, ATC
Oklahoma Center for Athletes
Oklahoma City, Oklahoma

Jerry Vannatta, MD
Associate Professor of Medicine
Department of Internal Medicine
University of Oklahoma
College of Medicine
Oklahoma City, Oklahoma

Kaye Wilkins, MD
Clinical Professor of Orthopaedics and
  Pediatrics
University of Texas
Health Sciences Center
San Antonio, Texas

David Yngve, MD
Associate Professor
Pediatric Orthopaedic Surgery
Childrens Hospital of Oklahoma
Oklahoma City, Oklahoma

Preface

The popularity of youth sports is at an all-time high and currently receives much media attention. Despite the popularity of the subject, scientific information about the pediatric athlete is limited. Children are not small adults and many of the studies on injury patterns, training techniques, and rehabilitation should not be extrapolated for use in pediatric athletes.

In November 1988, the American Academy of Orthopaedic Surgeons sponsored a seminar entitled "The Pediatric Athlete: Guidelines for Participation." This seminar brought together specialists from orthopaedics, pediatrics, psychology, exercise physiology, physical therapy, and education. The objective of the seminar was to review the available information about fitness, conditioning, patterns of injury, and rehabilitation in the pediatric athlete. We then hoped to summarize the factual information. Where no factual information or scientific validation was available, we hoped to reach consensual agreement. Thus, at the end of some sections are consensus statements developed at the seminar to provide the reader with the participants' perspective on these areas. This book is a collation of the information, both factual and consensual, presented at that meeting.

The sports science section contains information on the effects of aerobic and anaerobic conditioning in the pediatric athlete and the implications of this information for training. We wanted to know if there were sex and age differences and whether the recommended aerobic and anaerobic techniques could enhance performance.

We also sought to discover whether the pediatric athlete has a different dietary requirement from his or her peers. Information on weight control, dietary supplements, and fluid and electrolyte balance are also presented.

Another section considers guidelines for participation and medication in the child with chronic illness. The preparticipation evaluation is important, and standards for this evaluation are given. The use of drugs and ergogenic aids is outlined.

In the musculoskeletal injury section, we summarize specific injury patterns that occur in the pediatric athlete by anatomic area rather than by sport. In each category we have tried to determine whether there is a specific sport that affects a specific anatomic area. We wanted to know whether the injuries could be prevented by conditioning, rules changes, or protective equipment changes, and if there were any long-term consequences of the above injuries.

We have become increasingly aware that overuse syndromes are important in the skeletally immature patient. These were specifically addressed in the presentations on the osteochondroses, the response of the skeleton to repetitive stress, and stress fractures in children.

It appeared to us as well that there is little information about the role of rehabilitation in the pediatric athlete. We sought to discover whether there are any modalities that are known to be effective and to explore the role of protective equipment.

Youth sports organizations have evolved over the past 100 years and have reached a sophisticated level. Children are introduced to organized sports at a young age. In the section on Sport Psychology and Organization, we have moved out of the field of medicine, believing that persons involved in the care of pediatric athletes should have information about the structures that govern youth sports. The value of sports psychology is acknowledged in relation to the adult athlete, and recent attention has proved its merit in the pediatric athlete as well, as we have attempted to bring out. The section also discusses role models as an influence in the development of pediatric athletes.

This book is intended for use by the wide variety of individuals who are involved with pediatric athletes. It is hoped that it will point out areas in which little information is known and therefore stimulate research in these areas.

We wish to acknowledge the support and funding support of the American Academy of Orthopaedic Surgeons. We especially thank the Academy's committees on Pediatric Orthopaedics and Sports Medicine for their efforts in making this seminar and publication possible.

We are particularly grateful for the assistance of Marilyn L. Fox, PhD, Wendy O. Schmidt, and Mark W. Wieting of the Academy office for their work in producing this publication. We also thank the Academy's Karen M. Schneider for her help in organizing the seminar. Finally, we are indebted to Karen Barger for making many of the arrangements and for her assistance in organizing the seminar.

J. Andy Sullivan, M.D.
William A. Grana, M.D.

Table of Contents

Section One

Training

Chapter 1

Children and Exercise: A Physiologic Perspective

Frank A. Kulling, EdD

A recent federal document established national health objectives to be met by 1990, many of which were directed toward youth.[1] Understanding a child's capacity for exercise is important as more children begin to exercise. This chapter will focus on those physiologic variables that determine "health-related fitness."[2]

Maximum oxygen uptake (VO_2 max) is perhaps the most important physiologic variable, since it requires the integrated functioning of the cardiovascular, pulmonary, and musculoskeletal systems.[3] In this area, Bar-Or[4] reviewed 19 studies involving almost 4,000 boys and girls 6 to 18 years old and found that reported weight-adjusted values for VO_2 max ranged from 35 to 60 mL/kg/min.[4] This compared favorably with results for adults.[5] Values for boys remained constant throughout the age range. Values for girls were generally lower than those for boys and declined after the age of 11 or 12 years,[4] perhaps because of increasing female adiposity associated with the maturation process.

In addition to VO_2 max, the anaerobic threshold is often used as a measure of aerobic or endurance potential, since it represents the upper limits of exercise intensity that can be sustained for prolonged periods.[6] When Cooper and associates[7] tested 109 boys and girls from 6 to 17 years old, the mean anaerobic threshold was 58% of VO_2 max. Davis and associates[8] found the mean anaerobic threshold of college men during treadmill exercise to be 58.6% of VO_2 max.

These studies seem to indicate that children are the equal of adults with respect to aerobic capacity. Daniels and associates,[9] however, found that 10-year-old boys expend 26% more energy than 18-year-olds when running. Thus, it seems that children experience a higher metabolic cost than adults for some endurance activities.

During a single exercise session, children exhibit lower stroke volumes than adults at all levels of exercise. This is largely compensated for by higher heart, oxygen extraction, and ventilation rates during exercise.[4,10]

When children "train" in endurance activities, performance is likely to improve but there may be no concomitant improvement in physiologic measures such as VO_2 max.[11,12] Rowland[13] found that VO_2 max increased when endurance exercise components corresponded to adult prescriptions. Kobayashi and associates[10] found that the greatest increase in aerobic capacity occurred during the periods of most rapid growth. Some investigators think that "geometric" and "dimensional" analyses should be used to evaluate pediatric aerobic capacity.[14] Studies have found that children respond to aerobic training with increased physical work capacity,[15] increased left ventricular mass,[16] and decreased submaximal heart rate.[12]

Although children may compare favorably with adults in endurance-related characteristics, they are less able to perform anaerobically, even when weight-adjusted measures are considered.[4] This anaerobic inferiority is not explained by differences in muscle cell morphology, since children possess fiber-type distribution ratios similar to those of adults.[17] Levels of creatine phosphate in resting muscle, adenosine triphosphate, and glycogen are also similar in both adults and children.[18] During exercise, however, children cannot utilize glycogen as efficiently as adults.[4] The fact that carbohydrates, particularly in the form of muscle glycogen, are the almost exclusive fuel source for anaerobic activity,[19] could explain the reduced anaerobic capacity of children. The biochemical harbinger may be limited phosphofructokinase activity, a key enzyme in the glycolytic reaction process.[4]

Although children cannot emulate adults in anaerobic activities, this may not be especially detrimental, particularly during activity transition. When the intensity of an activity increases significantly, immediate energy demands must often be met anaerobically. Cardiorespiratory adjustments may take some time, creating an oxygen "deficit." During submaximal exercise, however, a new oxygen "steady state" is achieved with aerobic pathways adequate for energy demands.[6] The time between the creation of the oxygen deficit and achievement of a new steady state is significantly less for children than for adults[20]; therefore, children do not have to rely as heavily on anaerobic pathways during activity transition.

Body composition measures are difficult to assess, because this variable is highly age- and sex-specific. There are few acceptable methods for comparing children with adults. An analysis of flexibility shows that girls are more flexible than boys and that young children are more flexible than adults.[21]

Investigators routinely find that muscle strength gains parallel growth, with maximum results reported somewhere during early adulthood. However, strength expressed per unit area of muscle tissue is similar for adults and for children of both sexes.[6] Additionally, children's muscle strength increases in response to the same relative overloads found to be effective for adults.[4]

During walking and running, children produce more metabolic heat than adults do.[4] Although children have a higher sweat gland density than adults, they produce less sweat to dissipate heat.[22] Additionally, children do not acclimatize to heat as quickly[23] or experience the effects of exercise as intensely as adults.[24] Since children experience increased ventilation rates,[10] they may be at increased risk from atmospheric pollutants during exercise. Finally, children recover from strenuous activity more rapidly than adults.[4]

Summary

"Health-related" physiologic variables[2] in children must be examined to determine the applicability and efficacy of exercise in a pediatric population. When weight-adjusted VO_2 max and proportional anaerobic threshold measures are used to indicate cardiopulmonary potential, children appear to be the equals of their adult counterparts.[4-8] Children have, however, demonstrated relative metabolic inefficiency in some endurance-related tasks and, therefore, are usually unable to perform at levels considered "normal" for adults.[9] During a single exercise session, children display physiologic responses similar to adults.[4,10]

Anaerobically, children are definitely inferior to adults, even when weight-adjusted comparisons are considered.[4] Their impaired glycolytic capabilities are a result of limited phosphofructokinase activity.[4] Children cannot be expected, therefore, to produce as much relative power as adults. However, this limitation may not be significant during submaximal activity transitions (from lower to higher intensities), since children reach a steady state more rapidly than adults.[20]

It is difficult to compare body composition measures of children and adults, since the variables are age- and sex-specific. Young children are more flexible than adults and girls are more flexible than boys.[21] In hot humid environments, children are at increased risk for heat-related illnesses because they take longer to acclimatize,[23] experience the effects of exercise less intensely,[24] produce more heat, and dissipate it more slowly than adults.[22] When children exercise in a polluted atmospheric environment, they may be at risk because their ventilatory rates exceed adult values.[10]

Exercise can benefit children in most of the same performance and physiologic ways documented for adults.[4,11-13,15,16]

References

1. U.S. Department of Health and Human Services: *Promoting Health/Preventing Disease: Objectives For The Nation.* US Government Printing Office, 1980.
2. Bar-Or O: A commentary to children and fitness: A public health perspective. *Res Q* 1987;58:304-307.
3. Wasserman, et al: *Principles of Exercise Testing and Interpretation.* Philadelphia, Lea & Febiger, 1987.
4. Bar-Or O: *Pediatric Sports Medicine for the Practitioner: From Physiologic Principles to Clinical Applications.* New York, Springer-Verlag, 1983.
5. Cooper KH: *The Aerobics Way.* New York, M Evans and Co, 1977.
6. DeVries H: *Physiology of Exercise for Physical Education and Athletics,* ed 4. Dubuque, Wm C Brown, 1986.

7. Cooper DM, Weiler-Ravell D, Whipp BJ, et al: Aerobic parameters of exercise as a function of body size during growth in children. *J Appl Physiol* 1984; 56:628-634.

8. Davis JA, Vodak P, Wilmore JH, et al: Anaerobic threshold and maximal aerobic power for three modes of exercise. *J Appl Physiol* 1976;41:544-550.

9. Daniels J, Oldridge N, Nagle F, et al: Differences and changes in Vo_2 among young runners 10 to 18 years of age. *Med Sci Sports* 1978;10:200-203.

10. Kobayashi K, Kitamura K, Miura M, et al: Aerobic power as related to body growth and training in Japanese boys: A longitudinal study. *J Appl Physiol* 1978;44:666-672.

11. Daniels J, Oldridge N: Changes in oxygen consumption of young boys during growth and running training. *Med Sci Sports* 1971;3:161-165.

12. Stewart KJ, Gutin B: Effects of physical training on cardiorespiratory fitness in children. *Res Q* 1976;47:110-120.

13. Rowland TW: Aerobic response to endurance training in prepubescent children: A critical analysis. *Med Sci Sports Exerc* 1985;17:493-497.

14. Asmussen E, Heebøll-Nielsen K: A dimensional analysis of physical performance and growth in boys. *J Appl Physiol* 1955;7:593-603.

15. Vaccaro P, Clarke DH: Cardiorespiratory alterations in 9 to 11 year old children following a season of competitive swimming. *Med Sci Sports* 1978;10:204-207.

16. Geenen SL, Gilliam TB, Crowley D, et al: Echocardiographic measures in 6 to 7 year old children after an 8 month exercise program. *Am J Cardiol* 1982; 49:1990-1995.

17. Bell RD, MacDougall JD, Billeter R, et al: Muscle fiber types and morphometric analysis of skeletal muscle in six-year-old children. *Med Sci Sports Exerc* 1980;12:28-31.

18. Eriksson BO: Muscle metabolism in children: A review. *Acta Paediatr Scand* 1980;283(suppl):20-28.

19. Brooks G, Fahey T: *Fundamentals of Human Performance.* New York, Macmillan, 1987.

20. Macek M, Vavra J: The adjustment of oxygen uptake at the onset of exercise: A comparison between prepubertal boys and young adults. *Int J Sports Med* 1980;1:75-77.

21. Phillips M, Bockwalter C, Denman C, et al: Analysis of results from the Kraus-Weber Test of minimum muscular fitness in children. *Res Q* 195 26:314-323.

22. Bar-Or O: Climate and the exercising child: A review. *Int J Spo s Med* 1980; 1:53-65.

23. Wagner JA, Robinson S, Tzankoff SP, et al: Heat tolerance and acclimatization to work in the heat in relation to age. *J Appl Physiol* 1972;33:616-622.

24. Bar-Or O: Age-related changes in exercise perception, in Borg G (ed): *Physical Work and Effort.* Oxford, Pergamon Press, 1977.

Chapter 2

Endurance Training of the Pediatric Athlete

Ronald A. Ratliff, PhD

Introduction

The increased participation of young athletes in organized youth sports and their interest in top-level competition necessitate a better understanding of children's physical training. Proper physical training may enhance sport performance capabilities and help the young athlete gain the full benefits of athletic training and competition.[1]

In sports, the term "training" refers to a long-term, specific exercise regimen that emphasizes improving a particular performance capability. Endurance training, therefore, refers to systematic and regular participation in exercises designed to enhance endurance. A realistic goal in designing an endurance training program is to increase the athlete's fatigue-resistance capability during prolonged sports participation. Fatigue affects performance skills and capabilities whenever the nature or demand of the sport activity exceeds the endurance capacity of the athlete. Sports such as distance running, for instance, call for prolonged periods of exercise at rather high intensities; sports such as soccer call for repetitive, intermittent periods of high-intensity exercise with only minimal periods of rest and recovery. Young athletes competing in either aerobic (endurance) or anaerobic (power) sports can benefit from endurance training.

Significance of Endurance Training in Children

A recent statement by the American College of Sports Medicine[2] indirectly supports at least modest levels of endurance training in children by saying physical fitness programs are important in the healthy development of children. The statement recommends that children engage in 20 to 30 minutes of vigorous activity each day to develop and maintain the ability to meet the physical demands of living and to promote optimal health.

Bar-Or[3] offered another significant application of endurance training programs for children—rehabilitation. Endurance training after recovery from injury or illness may help a child to return to a normal level of physical functioning more rapidly and safely.

Endurance training to enhance sports performance, however, can be distinguished from training designed to improve physical fitness or to rehabilitate the child recovering from illness or injury. Although the general principles and dimensions of endurance training can be applied to programs for nonathletes, specific goals are included in the design of training programs for athletes. A greater emphasis is placed on specificity, increasing levels of graduated and progressive overload, and tailoring the training program to match sport requirements with the child's capabilities. Other important considerations include tapering or increasing exercise levels for optimal performance and coordinating seasonal variations in intensity, duration, and frequency.

The few studies of training in children have produced contradictory findings because of their failure to control for the effects of the child's growth, maturation, and physical-activity patterns.[4,5] Of interest, however, is the recognition that the intense training and competition considered normal for the adult athlete are not generally recommended for the young athlete.[6] For now, since no substantial information on the physiologic or psychologic risks to children from systematic overloading of the body in endurance training is available, it seems reasonable that levels of training for optimal sports performance in children should be substantially less than those recommended for adults.

Determinants of Endurance Performance

A recent review by Sjödin and Svedenhag[7] linked specific physiologic determinants with successful marathon running, a prolonged endurance event. These determinants are maximum oxygen uptake (VO_2 max), economy of motion, the anaerobic or lactate threshold, the percent of utilization of VO_2 max, and fuel supply and utilization.

Economy of motion is the amount of energy (measured as VO_2 max, or oxygen uptake) required to elicit a given amount of work. An athlete's anaerobic or lactate threshold occurs with the onset of blood lactate accumulation at a specific level (for instance, 4 mmol). It is often described as a percentage of VO_2 max. Percentage utilization of VO_2 max is the percentage of maximal oxygen uptake utilized at a specified submaximal level of work. Fuel supply and utilization are factors because the onset of fatigue from prolonged endurance events is related to depletion of muscle glycogen. Thus, preferential use of fats spares these carbohydrate reserves.

Training programs that focus on these determinants of endurance performance can reasonably be expected to be more successful. The training experience and laboratory data used to develop these determinants, however, are almost entirely derived from studies of adult athletes. As discussed in Chapter 1, because the response and adaptation patterns of children to endurance training can be distinguished from those observed in adults, the data do not prove conclusively that physiologic determinants are as important in children as they are in adults.

Trainability of Endurance Performance in Children

As noted in Chapter 1, training does not substantially improve VO_2 max in children, when expressed in relation to body weight. There are other determinants of endurance capacity that may contribute to the athlete's enhanced performance with training. It has been suggested that training improves performance in children by producing either better economy of motion or greater anaerobic capacity.[8] The few studies of alterations in economy of motion or anaerobic capacities in children do not demonstrate how children improve performance with training. It has also been suggested that endurance athletes who "push themselves harder" without overtraining, are more successful.[6] Bar-Or[8] concluded that, although prepubescent children are trainable, a question remains regarding their ability to improve their aerobic power. He further stated that VO_2 max may not be a valid criterion of maximal aerobic power. Noakes[9] suggested that specific dimensions of muscle contractility power, which may be independent of tissue oxygen deficiency, could be a better explanation of maximal aerobic athletic performance. In this context he cited research by Reybrouck and associates[10] that explains the potential importance to endurance performance of the lactate threshold and percentage utilization of VO_2 max determinants. There is some evidence that the effect of endurance training is greatest when changes in height (peak height velocity) are greatest.[11]

To resolve the questions that abound regarding the trainability of children, systematic, longitudinal research is needed. Investigators must attempt to control for the effects of growth, maturation, and physical-activity habits that are known to influence research findings. Further, factors such as a child's less efficient economy of motion, increased ratio of surface area to body mass, and apparent immaturity of specific metabolic (exergonic) pathways must be carefully evaluated if the sport scientist is to better understand the role of training in children.[1,3,12]

Endurance Training Guidelines

Children differ from adults physiologically, anatomically, and psychologically. These differences should be taken into account in interpreting and designing children's training programs. The apparent differences in trainability between children and adults demonstrate that children are not "miniature" adults. Issues within these areas merit more research, including determination of the earliest age at which intense endurance training should be initiated. Also, the potential risks associated with vigorous endurance training of the pediatric athlete have not been adequately measured. Despite the apparent limitations of applying to children physiologic training principles derived from work with adults, conventional wisdom has accepted this leap, albeit with reservations.[3,6,13] More complete and technical discussions of the principles and dimensions of physical training are available elsewhere.[6,14,15]

A training program must take intensity, duration, and frequency into account. The type or mode of activity determines what specific neuromuscular coordinative movement patterns should be included in the program. Cross-training does not seem to be associated with achieving optimal performance in the more basic sports such as running, cycling, and swimming.[14,16]

Adaptation results from progressive overloading. As intensity, duration, and frequency of training increase, specific adaptation to the imposed demands occurs. In general, prolonged, primarily aerobic exercise is used to improve endurance performance, whereas high-intensity, short-interval exercise develops anaerobic or short-term power performance. However, specialized anaerobic training can augment aerobic training by enhancing selected determinants of endurance.

An effective, long-term training program must meet specific performance goals, but the program should also be a positive and enjoyable experience for the child. Because children do not normally seek prolonged, monotonous training activities, a child's program should involve more "play" than the adult athlete's program. The degree of overload must be substantially less than that known to promote top performance in adults.

Planning a Training Program   The design of an endurance training program is based on the intensity, duration, frequency, perceived effort, and repetition of exercise.

Intensity   Intensity of endurance training is commonly determined by measuring VO_2 max or heart rate. The endurance training session is described as a specified percentage of VO_2 max or the maximum heart rate. A minimum-intensity threshold is necessary to elicit beneficial adaptive changes in the aerobic system. Although no specific data are available regarding children, these values for adults are 50% to 60% of VO_2 max or about 60% to 70% of the maximum heart rate.

The anaerobic system begins to gain an increasingly dominant role in meeting energy demands at an exercise intensity of about 70% to 80% of VO_2 max or 80% to 90% of the maximum heart rate. This serves as an upper limit for the aerobic training zone. A sound training program to enhance optimally endurance performance should also include some anaerobic exercise with an appropriate overload stimulus.[16]

A perception of effort termed "perceived exertion" can also be used to gauge intensity of effort.[15] This psychological rating of perceived exertion on a scale of 6 through 20 has been shown to be a reliable and valid indicator of heart rate, percentage of VO_2 max, and lactate threshold.[17] Interestingly, children seem to rate exercise at a specified physiologic strain somewhat lower on the scale than do older persons.[3]

Duration   Duration refers to the length of a training session. Endurance training may consist of one continuous workout or several repetitive sessions at intervals. As duration increases, the intensity of effort must decrease if participation in the training session is to continue. In the design of a training program, there is no optimal duration, although health-fitness prescriptions generally recommend exercise durations of approximately 15 to 40 minutes or more.[18] The duration of a workout depends on several factors, such as the specific sport or activity involved and the intensity of the training sessions. Because children do not respond well to prolonged, monotonous exercise efforts, their workouts should consist of repetitions rather than long, continuous sessions. Although there are no physiologic data to explain the phenomenon, children are often more willing than adults to begin new exercise sessions after a previous "perceived" all-out or almost all-out session.[8]

Frequency   No particular frequency of exercise sessions per week is considered optimal. Guidelines generally recommend a minimum of two or three to a maximum of four or five exercise sessions per week.[18] Because frequency interacts with intensity and duration, increasing or decreasing frequency often means that intensity or duration must be decreased or increased, respectively, to achieve the same training overload. Costill[16] stated that the factors that should determine the number of training sessions per week are the stage of training, the individual's tolerance to training, and the pace and distance of training. Individual differences in training tolerance are determined by the athlete's ability to recover, that is, the amount of rest needed between training sessions. Rapidly growing children probably require at least several days without training each week, although, as with intensity and duration, there has been no systematic effort to determine the optimal training frequency for children.

It is unlikely that an optimal training regimen can be prescribed for the pediatric athlete. Common sense suggests that a child's endurance training program be conservative and easily tolerated—physiologically, psychologically, and clinically.

Seasonal variations should also be considered. Preseason training should de-emphasize strain (intensity on the body's physiologic systems) and emphasize a progressive increase in volume (duration). As a sport's competitive season approaches, increased emphasis should be placed on progressive increases in intensity overload.

Specific Endurance Training Techniques   Wells and Pate[14] recently discussed the physiologic rationales and components of four training programs that have proven to be effective in adults. These are summarized in Table 1. These programs reflect the interdependent nature of intensity, duration, and frequency. The data also show that as training progresses from low-intensity to high-intensity regimens there is greater specific adaptation of the anaerobic energy systems and related performance components. It is important to re-emphasize when developing a training program for children, that they are not miniature adults. Additionally, the amount of training should be substantially less in volume and intensity for children.

Table 1. Summary of Training Techniques for Endurance Performance

	Long Slow Distance	Aerobic Interval	Pace/Tempo	Anaerobic Interval
I	65 to 70% VO_{2max} 75 to 80% MHR (Steady state VO_2)	70 to 80% VO_{2max} 80 to 90% MHR (Slightly less than race pace or below lactate threshold)	80 to 95% VO_{2max} 90 to 95% MHR (Slightly above race pace and/or lactate threshold)	95 to 120% VO_{2max} 95 to 100% MHR (Above lactate threshold)
D	> 1 Hour	5–15 Minutes (Depends on performance goal)	3–10 Minutes (Depends on performance goal)	30 Sec–4 Min
F	~1/week	~3–4/week	~1–2/week	~1/week REPS: 5–20
RPE	10,11,12 Fairly light	13,14,15 Somewhat hard	15,16,17 Hard to very hard	18,19,20 Very, very hard

I—Intensity; D—Duration; F—Frequency; RPE—Rating of Perceived Exertion; REPS—Repetitions.
Adapted with permission from Wells CL, and Pate RR: Training for performance of prolonged exercise, in Lamb DR, (ed): *Perspectives in Exercise Science and Sports Medicine: Prolonged Exercise.* Indianapolis, Benchmark Press, 1988, vol 1, pp 357-391.

Warming Up and Down Warming up should begin with stretching exercises and progress to activities similar to those that will be included in the training session. The rationale is that by warming up the young athlete is better prepared for the workout. Although the scientific evidence is unclear, it seems reasonable that warming up permits some physiologic adjustment to the energy demands of hard exercise. It may also help reduce the risk of injury.

A warming-down period after the training session is commonly recommended, but again without a clear scientific rationale. However, the rate at which lactate is removed from the blood is higher during a physically active recovery than during an inactive recovery.[19] This factor may be of particular interest to trainers trying to hasten recovery between exercise intervals during pace-tempo or anaerobic-interval training.

Sport-Specific Training Programs

The training guidelines and general training techniques discussed can be applied to both distance running and predominantly anaerobic sports such as soccer and basketball. The programs presented are based on three criteria: proven success in practice, a reasonable match between sport performance goals and training procedures, and available knowledge concerning physiologic response and adaptation patterns.

Elite Distance Runners Training programs should be designed so that high-volume training is used during the off-season and early in the season and high-intensity training is used later in the season.[6] The athlete should begin with sustained, moderate-intensity or long, slow (less than race pace) runs.[20] As the season progresses, the emphasis should shift to pace-tempo and/or anaerobic-interval training, with the athlete running several times a week at faster than race pace.[14]

Three-week cycles of light, moderate, and hard workouts provide variations in stress and overload and permit specific training of different systems.[16] As intensity increases, duration should be reduced. For peak performance during races, a one- to two-week period of gradually decreasing training (about one-third of the normal daily mileage) is recommended before major competitions.[21]

During high-volume training, adult elite runners often run 40 to 80 miles per week.[16] The prepubescent athlete should probably run no more than 14 to 30 miles per week.

Anaerobic Sports   Endurance training can be useful for the young athlete participating in a sport that is primarily anaerobic in nature. Such sports include soccer, basketball, and tennis. Training the aerobic system should provide the following performance benefits: increased aerobic reserve capacity (working at a smaller percentage of VO_2 max); enhanced recovery after an intense workout or prolonged intense intermittent activity; and altered fuel utilization patterns at a given submaximal workload that conserve muscle and liver glycogen reserves. In addition, preseason endurance training can provide a more gradual acclimation to training stresses, thereby better preparing the musculoskeletal framework for the increased demands of an intense competitive season. Among the seasonal components of a specific endurance training program for anaerobic sports are preseason volume training (long, slow distance runs and aerobic-interval training three times per week), preseason and early-season volume and high-intensity training (aerobic-interval and pace-tempo training two or three times per week), and in-season high-intensity training.

In all training programs, the overriding concern should be to increase stress gradually so that the body will adapt to the demands imposed by competition. In training to enhance endurance performance for an anaerobic sport, the pediatric athlete is probably best served by training concentrated somewhat on the movement patterns utilized in that sport or activity. However, training should not ignore the need to exercise other muscle groups. Some generalized or cross-training is probably necessary to avoid injury and to achieve muscular balance.[22]

Special Endurance Training Considerations

There are a number of special considerations associated with the development and implementation of an optimal endurance training program for young athletes. These include overtraining, the effects of interruption of training on performance, the application of tapering techniques to achieve peak performance, the benefits of cross-training, special constraints imposed by climatic conditions (heat, cold, high altitude), and the role played by the medical team monitoring the program.

Summary

The pediatric athlete can benefit from a properly designed endurance training program. Although most training programs for children are based primarily on research done on adults, there are unique characteristics that distinguish children's responses and adaptations to training from those observed in adults. Scientists and coaches currently believe that the general principles and dimensions of an endurance training program for adults can be applied to a program for children. Nonetheless, these distinguishing characteristics should be taken into account when programs are designed. Training regimens should be conservative and the program should emphasize "play" and individual performance goals. It is important that the young athlete be medically examined before participating in a vigorous endurance training program.

References

1. Bailey DA, Mirwald RL: The effects of training on the growth and development of the child, in Malina RM (ed): *Young Athletes: Biological, Psychological and Educational Perspectives*. Champaign, Human Kinetics, 1988, pp 33-48.
2. American College of Sports Medicine: Opinion statement on physical fitness in children and youth. *Med Sci Sport Exerc* 1988;20:422-423.
3. Bar-Or O: *Pediatric Sports Medicine for the Practitioner: From Physiologic Principles to Clinical Applications*. New York, Springer, 1983.
4. Rowland TW, Green GM: Physiological responses to treadmill exercise in females: Adult-child differences. *Med Sci Sport Exerc* 1988;20:474-478.
5. Cunningham DA, Paterson DH, Blimkie CJ: The development of the cardiorespiratory system with growth and physical activity, in Boileau RA (ed): *Advances in Pediatric Sport Sciences*. Champaign, Human Kinetics, 1984, pp 85-119.
6. Wilmore JH, Costill DL: *Training for Sport and Activity*. Dubuque, Iowa, Wm C Brown, 1988.
7. Sjödin B, Svedenhag J: Applied physiology of marathon running. *Sports Med* 1985;2:83-99.
8. Bar-Or O: Importance of differences between children and adults for exercise testing and exercise prescription, in Skinner JS (ed): *Exercise Testing and Exercise Prescription for Special Cases*. Philadelphia, Lea & Febiger, 1987, pp 49-65.
9. Noakes TM: Implications of exercise testing for prediction of athletic performance: A contemporary perspective. *Med Sci Sport Exerc* 1988;20:319-330.
10. Reybrouck T, Ghesquiere J, Cattaert A, et al: Ventilatory thresholds during short- and long-term exercise. *J Appl Physiol* 1983;55:1694-1700.
11. Robayashi K, Kitamura K, Miura M, et al: Aerobic power as related to body growth and training in Japanese boys: A longitudinal study. *J Appl Physiol* 1978;44:666-672.
12. Rowland W, Auchinachie JA, Keenan TJ, et al: Physiologic responses to treadmill running in adult and prepubertal males. *Int J Sports Med* 1987;8:292-297.
13. Martens R, Christina RW, Harvey JS, et al: *Coaching Young Athletes*. Champaign, Human Kinetics, 1981.

14. Wells CL, Pate RR: Training for performance of prolonged exercise, in Lamb DR (ed): *Perspectives in Exercise Science and Sports Medicine: Prolonged Exercise.* Indianapolis, Benchmark Press, 1988, vol 1, pp 357-391.

15. Noble BJ: *Physiology of Exercise and Sport.* St. Louis, Times Mirror/Mosby, 1986.

16. Costill DL: *Inside Running: Basis of Sports Physiology.* Indianapolis, Benchmark Press, 1986.

17. Hanson P: Clinical exercise testing, in Blair S, Painter P, Pate RR (eds): *Resource Manual for Guidelines for Exercise Testing and Prescription.* Philadelphia, Lea & Febiger, 1988, pp 205-222.

18. American College of Sports Medicine: *Guidelines for Graded Exercise Testing and Exercise Prescription,* ed 2. Philadelphia, Lea & Febiger, 1980.

19. Hermansen L, Stensvold I: Production and removal of lactate during exercise in man. *Acta Physiol Scand* 1972; 86:191-201.

20. Daniels J, Fitts R, Sheehan G: *Conditioning for Distance Running.* New York, John Wiley & Sons, 1978.

21. Costill DL, King DS, Thomas R, et al: Effects of reduced training on muscular power in swimmers. *Phys Sports Med* 1985;13:94-101.

22. Sharkey BJ: Specificity of exercise, in Blair S, Painter P, Pate RR (eds): *Resource Manual for Guidelines for Exercise Testing and Prescription.* Philadelphia, Lea & Febiger, 1988 pp 55-61.

Chapter 3

Strength Training

Lyle J. Micheli, MD

Incorporating strength training into the overall training regimen of elite and recreational athletes has gained widespread acceptance and has even been extended to the management of certain adult disease states, such as osteoporosis.[1-3] In athletes, strength training can enhance performance and help prevent injury.[4-6] Strength training has had positive effects on athletic performance and motor skills in adult male and adult female athletes. Recent studies of strength training in adolescents of both sexes have also shown positive effects in sports as varied as distance running, gridiron football, and gymnastics.[1,7]

The use of strength training in younger athletes (those in Tanner I or II stages of development) is still controversial.[8-10] The controversy focuses on three areas: (1) Are children capable of making significant strength gains and increases in muscle mass in response to resistive strength training? (2) Do these gains in strength improve athletic performance or increase the resistance of the child's tissue to injury? (3) Do children have an unacceptable risk of injury from resistive strength training that negates any potential benefits from the technique?

Since some confusion exists about the terms used in strength training and weight lifting, it is useful to begin by defining them. Strength training is the use of resistance methods to increase one's ability to exert or resist force.[11] The training may use free weights, body weight, machines, or other training devices to attain this goal. To be effective, the training sessions must include timely progressions in intensity, which impose sufficient demands to stimulate strength gains greater than those of normal development. Resistive training is any method or form used to resist, overcome, or bear force. Weight training is the use of barbells, dumbbells, or machine-type apparatus as resistance. Weight lifting and power lifting are competitive sports. Olympic weight lifting includes the techniques of Olympic snatch, squat, and clean-and-jerk, while power lifting involves competition in bench press and dead-lift.

Effects of Resistance Strength Training in the Child

A number of studies suggest that prepubescent children, when placed on a properly designed strength-training program, can increase voluntary strength.[10,12-14] Most of these studies used resistive weight training as a technique for enhancing strength, while several used isometric contractions, wrestling drills, or pneumatic machines. In the Vrijens study, published in 1978, a group of 16 boys with a mean age of 10.4 years did isotonic weight training three days a week for eight weeks.[15] They performed eight to 12 repetitions of each of eight exercises. The load corresponded to 70% of one repetition maximum (1 RM) in this study. These prepubescent boys failed to make significant increases in four of the six strength tests, but their back and abdominal strength increased significantly. A similar group of adolescent boys, with a mean age of 16.7 years, made significant strength gains in all areas.

Pfeiffer and Francis[16] compared repetitive strength training in prepubescent, pubescent, and postpubescent males in 1986. Weight training, using free weights and weight stack machines, was done three days a week for eight weeks. Nine exercises were performed in three sets of 50%, 75%, and 100% of the 10 RM. Strength was measured as peak torque of concentric contractions and at joint angle velocities of 30 and 120 degrees per second. Their findings suggest the greatest increase in relative strength occurred among the prepubescent males, contradicting the Vrijens study.

Sewall and Micheli[10] studied boys and girls 10 to 11 years old. This study involved resistive strength training of knee extension, chest press, and rowing, three days a week for nine weeks, with three sets of ten repetitions at 50%, 80%, and 100% of the 10 RM. All strength modality studies increased, except for knee flexion, and shoulder flexion showed a significant increase when compared with control groups. Weltman and associates'[17] studies on 16 prepubescent boys 6 to 11 years old used hydraulic resistance three days a week for 14 weeks. The training group made significantly greater increases in strength than the control group.

Rians and associates[12] also found significant strength gains in a group of prepubescent boys who used circuit weight training over a 12-week period.

Clarke and associates[18] studied 23 prepubescent boys who underwent three months of wrestling practices. In comparison to the control group, the wrestling group had significant increases in dips, chin-ups, and isometric leg-press strength.

Three recent studies have been published in abstract form. In 1984, McGovern[19] reported on 42 girls and boys in grades four through six involved in circuit weight training for 12 weeks. This group showed significant strength gains, measured by the training exercises, when compared with the control group. Servedio and associates[13] studied 44 boys and girls who did 30 minutes of calisthenics and exercises with stretch tubing, hand weights, and ball, three days a week for 12 weeks. They noted a significant increase in hand-grip strength, flexed arm hang, and pull-ups, but isometric elbow flexion extension did not increase.

Sale[20] reported on 13 prepubescent boys involved in weight training for 20 weeks. These children did three sets of 10 to 12 RM for ten weeks and five to seven RM for ten weeks. Strength was measured as the 1 RM on the training equipment, as well as peak torque on isokinetic and isometric dynamometers. The training group made significant increases in all but isometric knee extension. These studies show convincing evidence that prepubescent children on a properly designed strength-training program are indeed capable of making strength gains.

Prevention of Injury

Some evidence suggests that a progressive strength-training program can strengthen tissue and decrease the rate of injury to musculoskeletal tissue, including ligaments, in adolescents. However, no study of this type has yet been done for prepubescents,[5] nor has there been a study on the relative risk or danger of strength training in the prepubescent. Several studies specifically asked if strength training was safe for the prepubescent athlete. They found no increased rate of injury in carefully supervised strength-training programs.[12,21-27]

Possible long-term deleterious effects from strength training are of concern. There is increased evidence that repetitive impact trauma in certain specific sports, such as gymnastics, can cause growth-plate arrest. In addition, a study from Japan[28] suggested that children involved in long-term heavy labor appear to have a stunting of growth above and beyond other factors, such as nutrition. Again, a properly designed program emphasizing high levels of resistive training might be valuable for modern children who are deprived of musculoskeletal stress in their daily activities. The use of strength training as an exercise prescription is perfectly logical and consistent with the musculoskeletal deprivation sustained by these children today.[16,29,30] The obvious questions, of course, are, "How much is enough? How much is too much?" Children's reactions to exercise merit careful attention.

References

1. Asmussen E: Growth in muscular strength and power, in Rarick LG (ed): *Physical Activity, Human Growth and Development*. New York, Academic Press, 1973, pp 60-79.
2. Clarke H: *Muscle Strength and Endurance in Man*. Englewood Cliffs, Prentice-Hall, 1966.
3. Wilmore JH: Alterations in strength, body composition, and anthropometric measurements consequent to a 10-week training program. *Med Sci Sports* 1974;5:133-138.
4. Bjorharaa BS: Flexibility and strength training considerations for young athletes. National Strength & Conditioning Assoc J 1982; Aug-Sept:62-64.
5. Cahill BR, Griffith EH: Effect of pre-season conditioning on the incidence and severity of high school football knee injuries. *Am J Sports Med* 1978;6:180-184.
6. DeLorme TL, Watkins AL: *Progressive Resistance Exercises: Techniques and Medical Applications*. New York, Appleton-Century-Crofts, 1951.
7. Blanksby G, Gregor J: Anthropometric strength and physical changes in male and female swimmers with progressive resistive training. *Aust J Sports Sci* 1981;1:3-6.
8. American Academy of Pediatrics: Weight training and weight lifting: Information for the pediatrician. *Phys Sportsmed* 1983;1:157-161.

9. Micheli LJ: Strength training in the young athlete, in Brown EW, Branta CE (eds): *Competitive Sports for Children and Youth*. Champaign, Human Kinetics.

10. Sewall L, Micheli LJ: Strength training for children. *J Pediatr Orthop* 1986;6:143-146.

11. Duda M: Prepubescent strength training gains support. *Phys Sportsmed* 1986;14:157-161.

12. Rians CB, Weltman A, Cahill BR, et al: Strength training for prepubescent males: Is it safe? *Am J Sports Med* 1987;15:483-489.

13. Servedio FJ, Bartels RL, Hamlin RL: The effects of weight training using Olympic style lifts on various physiological variables in prepubescent boys. *Med Sci Sports Exerc* 1985;17:288.

14. Siegel JA, Camaione DN, Manfredi TG: Upper body strength training and prepubescent children. *Med Sci Sports Exerc* 1988;20(suppl):S53.

15. Vrijens J: Muscle strength development in the pre- and post-pubescent age. *Med Sport* 1978;11:152-158.

16. Pfeiffer RD, Francis RS: Effects of strength training on muscle development in prepubescent, pubescent, and postpubescent males. *Phys Sportsmed* 1986;14:134-143.

17. Weltman A, Janney C, Rians CB, et al: The effects of hydraulic resistance strength training in pre-pubertal males. *Med Sci Sports Exerc* 1986;18:629-638.

18. Clarke DH, Vaccaro P, Andresen NM: Physiological alterations in 7- to 9-year-old boys following a season of competitive wrestling. *Res Q Exerc Sport* 1984;55:318-322.

19. McGovern MB: Effects of circuit weight training on the physical fitness of prepubescent children. *Diss Abs Int* 1984;45:452A-453.

20. Sale DG: Neural adaptation in strength and power training, in Jones NL, McCartney N, McComas AJ (eds): *Human Muscle Power*. Champaign, Human Kinetics, 1986.

21. Brady TA, Cahill, BR, Bodnar L: Weight training-related injuries. *Am J Sports Med* 1982;10:1-5.

22. Jesse JP: Olympic weight lifting movements endanger adolescent weight lifters. *Phys Sportsmed* 1977;5:61-67.

23. Kulund DN, Dewey JB, Brubaker CE, et al: Olympic weight lifting injuries. *Phys Sportsmed* 1978:6:111-119.

24. Legwold G: Does lifting weights harm a prepubescent athlete? *Phys Sportsmed* 1982;10:141-144.

25. Mason TA: Is weight lifting deleterious to the spines of young people? *Br J Sports Med* 1970;5:54-56.

26. Ryan JR, Salciccioli GG: Fracture of the distal radial epiphysis in adolescent weightlifters. *Am J Sports Med* 1975;4:26-27.

27. Wilkins KE: The uniqueness of the young athlete: Musculoskeletal injuries. *Am J Sports Med* 1980;8:377-382.

28. Kato S, Ishiko T: Obstructive growth of children's bone due to excessive labor in remote countries, in Kato S (ed): *Proceedings of the International Congress of Sports Science*. Tokyo, University of Sport Science, 1984.

29. DeLorme TL, Ferris BG, Gallagher JR: Effect of progressive resistance exercise on muscle contraction time. *Arch Phys Med Rehabil* 1952;33:86-92.

30. Larson RL: Physical activity and the growth and development of bone and joint structures, in Rarick GL (ed): *Physical Activity, Human Growth and Development*. New York, Academic Press, 1973.

Chapter 4

Neuromuscular Training

Brian J. Sharkey, PhD

Introduction

Until recently, the pediatric athlete has been treated like a miniature adult. Faced with a lack of research on appropriate ways to train, coaches have used exercise prescriptions based on studies of and experience with more mature athletes. The young athlete is not a scaled-down adult, however, and responds differently to exercise and training.

For example, children are metabolically less efficient than adults, and require more oxygen (per kilogram of body weight) to run at a given pace. They exhibit lower anaerobic capabilities than older youths or adults, and their lactate levels in muscle and blood are lower. They have higher heart rates and lower stroke volumes during exertion and their respiratory apparatus seems less efficient. Thermoregulation is less effective since sweat rates are lower and the threshold for sweating is higher. Moreover, while children have a greater density of sweat glands, the adult gland produces 2.5 times as much sweat.[1]

These and other developmental or age-related differences between prepubescent children and young adults illustrate the need for systematic studies of the pediatric athlete to determine safe and effective exercise prescriptions. In the absence of these studies, coaches continue to use adult prescriptions, thereby risking short- and long-term consequences. Short-term consequences include illness or injury caused by overtraining, while long-term consequences include serious injury, burnout, and loss of interest.

Adaptations to Training

This section considers neuromuscular training techniques and explains how they should be modified to suit children. To avoid injury, training usually progresses from low-intensity aerobic work to high-intensity anaerobic effort.

But other issues also merit consideration. When should children begin competition (or training for competition)? What is the optimal time to start training and how can it be determined? What are the effects of improper or excessive training on future participation? And how can information on prudent exercise and training prescriptions be developed and disseminated?

Studies on adults support the principle of specificity of training. Regular aerobic exercise such as running leads to adaptations in aerobic enzymes and pathways in the muscle fibers used in the activity, while resistance training leads to increases in contractile protein. Endurance training produces peripheral effects, adaptations in and around the muscles, and then central effects, including changes in respiration, cardiac function, blood volume, and distribution of blood flow. In general, peripheral effects are more specific while central changes are more likely to transfer from one exercise to another. Evidence is lacking, however, on the effects of specificity of training for the pediatric athlete.

Aerobic Training In children, aerobic capacity (in liters) is considerably lower than in adults, primarily because of body size. Aerobic power (in ml per kilogram), on the other hand, is not deficient. Yet because they are not as efficient as adults, children work with a higher heart rate and a lower stroke volume to achieve the same cardiac output and stroke volume as adults. Despite these differences, little data exist to support modified aerobic exercise prescriptions. Training studies often fail to yield significant increases in aerobic power. Aerobic capacity (in liters) usually increases in proportion to body size, but oxygen intake in ml per kg of body weight does not. This finding is even more interesting when viewed in relation to performance improvements that may be caused by changes in body size.[2] Of course, improvements in neuromuscular skill and efficiency will contribute to enhanced performance in endurance events. For example, swimmers in training may show increases in aerobic power compared with their performance before training. All things considered, however, it seems unnecessary to place the pediatric athlete in serious endurance training programs.

On the other hand, apart from problems of efficiency and thermoregulation in hot climates, there does not seem to be an underlying physiologic factor making children less suitable than adults for prolonged, continuous activities.[3] A prudent approach could include moderate endurance training and competition. It may be that the repetitions of endurance training are more useful for increasing neuromuscular skill and efficiency in the prepubescent athlete, and that significant changes in peripheral and central factors await sexual maturity, the growth spurt, or some other biologic event.

Anaerobic Threshold The anaerobic threshold is the term coaches and athletes use for the lactate (or ventilatory) threshold. It marks the increase in blood lactate accumulation during exercise of increasing intensity. This threshold has been correlated to performance in endurance events such as the 10K run, and marks the maximal velocity that can be sustained.

As noted in Chapter 1, young athletes are less able to utilize muscle glycogen and to produce lactate than adults. Since threshold training involves training near the lactate threshold (or the threshold heart rate), it seems unnecessary to subject young athletes to this intense and demanding effort.[4] Coaches may want to use some threshold training to help athletes achieve relaxation at that level of exertion, but sustained long intervals, pace training, fartlek, and other approaches to improving the anaerobic threshold seem unnecessary. Moreover, such training may be inadvisable if it results in fatigue, burnout, or reduced interest in the sport.

Anaerobic Training   The anaerobic capabilities of children are lower than those of adults, even when expressed per unit of body weight (anaerobic power). Since anaerobic training of adults results in minimal changes, and since the rate of development of anaerobic capabilities is age-related, anaerobic interval training seems to have limited value for the pediatric athlete. It may be useful in developing neuromuscular skill, mechanical efficiency, and "psychological toughness," but excessive interval training at this stage could lead to injury and early burnout.[4,5]

Neuromuscular Training   Neuromuscular training affects two major areas: skill and efficiency (economy), and strength. Skill and efficiency are acquired through repeated movement patterns. With proper coaching, athletes become more skilled in the movements required. With this skill comes a dramatic reduction in the amount of energy used. It appears that motor skills and efficiency develop similarly in children, and that skill is more a function of practice than it is of age.[5]

Adults gain strength through a combination of neurogenic and myogenic adaptations. Neurogenic changes include improved recruitment of motor units, reduced inhibitions, and skill in the application of force. Myogenic adaptations include increased contractile proteins (actin and myosin), thickening of connective tissue, and, possibly, increases in short-term energy sources (creatine phosphate). Although children probably experience neurogenic changes, the evidence for myogenic changes in prepubescent athletes is lacking.[4,6]

Recent studies show that children are able to increase strength through resistance training.[7] Without the hormonal support necessary to increase muscle mass, children are less likely to increase muscle girth in a strength-training program. Although there is clear evidence that resistance training improves strength, muscle hypertrophy or increased lean body mass beyond that associated with normal growth is seldom seen. Hence, the training is largely neurogenic in nature.[4]

All prepubescent children respond similarly to training. Exercise prescriptions similar to those used for adults (three sets of six to ten repetitions, done three days each week) seem to yield significant increases in strength without injury. However, neurogenic changes in strength have not yet been related to performance in sport, nor is it clear how much strength is required for performance in a given sport. What is clear is that significant strength and muscle development depends on maturation and hormonal support. Muscle development is limited when the anabolic steroid testosterone is in short supply. Serum testosterone levels are not increased after training in prepubescent boys, as they are in the later stages of maturation.[8] Although sexual maturity gives men a hormonal advantage in strength development, women can experience muscle hypertrophy with sufficient training.

Implications

Prudent vs Proven Prescriptions   Without proven pediatric exercise prescriptions, coaches are forced to decide on a prudent course of action. The available evidence indicates that adult prescriptions for aerobic exercise can be used if extremes in exercise duration are avoided. High heat and humidity conditions should also be avoided because of the thermoregulatory limitations of children.[1]

Serious efforts to raise the anaerobic threshold seem destined to failure. Longer intervals can be used in children to enhance neuromuscular benefits, but fewer repetitions are necessary. Anaerobic training should be kept to the minimum required to develop skill, efficiency, and "acclimatization" to speed (relaxation, mental toughness).

Adult prescriptions for strength training may be used for children, but careful warm-up and proper lifting, with spotting and supervision, are necessary. The training apparatus should be scaled down to fit the pediatric athlete. It may be possible to achieve the neurogenic benefits of resistance training with lighter weights and more repetitions, thus reducing the risk of injury to the immature skeleton.

When Should Training for Competition Begin?   This question has several variations, such as: What is the optimal time for training in relation to age? Sexual maturation? Growth spurts? Other indicators? It is generally believed that when training begins too late in life the athlete is unlikely to reach full genetic potential. However, little empirical evidence exists to support or focus that assertion. Female gymnasts and swimmers begin early to master and develop neuromuscular skills and capabilities before menarche causes changes in body fat and in the ratio of strength to body weight that makes performance more difficult. Intense early training can even delay the onset of menarche by five months for each year of training.[9] Boys start later because they experience more success when they train during and after puberty.

Researchers have attempted to determine the optimal time for training, and have correlated improvements to growth spurt and sexual maturation. The peak height velocity has been used as one measure of the growth spurt. The peak for boys is at 13 to 14 years, whereas it occurs earlier (at 11 to 12 years) in girls. Although maximal aerobic power seems to spurt near the time of peak height velocity in boys, such a pattern has not been found in girls. Boys decline in motor performance during the growth spurt and begin a rebound about two years later.

There is little difference between preadolescent boys and girls in strength. Boys increase in strength from early childhood to peak height velocity, when strength development accelerates into the early 20s. Strength increases in young girls in a linear fashion up to the age of 15 years, and there is no evidence of an adolescent spurt.[6]

These findings do little to alter the prudent prescriptions offered earlier. For an individual to reach genetic potential, training may need to begin during the growth spurt. Although the standard deviation for peak height velocity is approximately one year, some youngsters experience a growth spurt as many as two or three years before (or after) the average age for their sex. Correlation with data on sexual maturation (such as the Tanner scale) would help avoid enormous errors in timing. Much more needs to be done before the appropriate age for training can be accurately predicted.

Effects of Early Training   Early training is not necessarily detrimental to health or performance. In fact, early training in girls, which has been associated with delayed menarche, has also been related to a lower incidence of reproductive cancers. However, strenuous training has also been associated with irregular cycles, amenorrhea, and osteoporosis.[9]

Early strenuous training may also be associated with eventual loss of interest or burnout. Although a girl's level of performance may decline as she adjusts to the increase in body fat that occurs after peak height velocity, several recent examples prove that women over 20 years old can achieve world-class swimming and gymnastics performances.[4]

Strenuous early training in boys is somewhat less common and considerably less successful. Serious training seems to have little value before the adolescent growth spurt. In countries where sports are part of a club system, prepubertal training focuses on skill development and fun. This often leads to extended involvement, with athletes participating in high-level training and competition well into their 30s. In the United States, however, youth sports programs serve as a farm system for schools. Here, early training and competition may serve to eliminate qualified athletes, especially those who experience a late adolescent growth spurt.

Summary

Pediatric athletes need exercise prescriptions and programs suited to their individual stages of development. Strenuous training before the growth spurt is usually less effective and more likely to lead to eventual loss of interest. Research is needed to develop appropriate exercise prescriptions, to assess the effects of training, and to determine the optimal time for training. Coaches who work with pediatric athletes need specific information and should be required to participate in coaching education programs.[4]

References

1. Bar-Or O: Importance of differences between children and adults for exercise testing and exercise prescription, in Skinner JS (ed): *Exercise Testing and Exercise Prescription for Special Cases: Theoretical Basis and Clinical Application*. Philadelphia, Lea & Febiger, 1987, pp 49-65.
2. Daniels J, Oldridge N: Changes in oxygen consumption in young boys during growth and running training. *Med Sci Sports* 1971;3:161-165.
3. Zwiren LD: Exercise prescription for children, in Blair S, Painter P, Pate RR, et al (eds): *Resource Manual for Guidelines for Exercise Testing and Prescription*. Philadelphia, Lea & Febiger, 1988, pp 309-314.
4. Sharkey B: When should children begin competing? A physiological perspective, in Weiss M, Gould D (eds): *Sports for Children and Youths*. Champaign, Human Kinetics, 1986, pp 51-54.
5. Vrijens J, Van Cauter C: Physical performance capacity and specific skills in young soccer players, in Binkhorst R, et al (eds): *Children and Exercise, XI*. Champaign, Human Kinetics, 1985, pp 285-292.
6. Beunen G, Malina R: Growth and physical performance relative to the timing of the adolescent spurt, in Pandolf K (ed): *Exercise and Sports Science Reviews*. New York, Macmillan, 1988, vol 16, pp 503-540.
7. Sewall L, Micheli LJ: Strength training for children. *J Pediatr Orthop* 1986;6:143-146.
8. Fahey TD, Del Valle-Zuris A, Oehlsen G, et al: Pubertal stage differences in hormonal and hematological responses to maximal exercise in males. *J Appl Physiol* 1979;46:823-827.
9. Frisch RE: Exercise, nutrition, puberty, and fertility: Delayed menarche and amenorrhea, in Borer KT, Edington DW, White TP (eds): *Frontiers of Exercise Biology*. Champaign, Human Kinetics, 1983, pp 198-213.

Chapter 5

Neurodevelopmental Milestones: When Is a Child Ready for Sports Participation?

Paul G. Dyment, MD

As more children compete in youth sports, parents turn to physicians and ask, "Should my 5-year-old son play ice hockey?" or, "Is my 8-year-old ready for tackle football?" The replies reflect the prejudices, biases, and upbringing of the physician, and few could survive scientific scrutiny.

An extensive computer-assisted review of the literature revealed no study that could answer such questions from a neurologic viewpoint. Trying to predict a child's readiness to learn a certain sport is hazardous. Even when the child is neurodevelopmentally ready, two other factors can negate that readiness: social development (does the child respond to the coach?) and cognitive level (can the child understand the instructions?). For example, at least 10% of all boys in elementary school have an attention-deficit disorder. The child may be developmentally ready to play baseball, but his attention span is so short that he gets bored playing in the outfield. If he also has motor-perceptual problems and cannot bat well, he may become an early drop-out. However, a wise coach might make him a catcher, a position where something is always happening, and where his attention can be sustained.

R.M. Malina defined "readiness" for sports as "the match between a child's level of growth, maturity, and development, and the task demands presented in competitive sports" (unpublished data). In this definition, growth refers to body size and composition, muscle strength, and aerobic power; maturity means skeletal age, pubertal age, chronological age, and level of proficiency in basic motor skills; and development includes social, emotional, and cognitive competence. Growth and maturity are basically biologic phenomena, genetic in origin. The development characteristics are biologic (cognitive competence), social (social competence), or both (emotional competence). Hence any approach to determining age-appropriateness for sports cannot be limited to levels of motor development, but must use a biosocial perspective.

Branta and associates[1] reviewed the data on age-related changes in the acquisition of motor skills, and found progressive improvement throughout childhood and adolescence. A gender difference appears at puberty. Girls reach a plateau or actually decline in their ability to perform certain skills, such as the flexed-arm hang, timed sit-ups, and leg lifts. Boys continue to improve in those skills requiring strength, power, and endurance. Bodie[2] studied ball-handling skills (dribbling, catching, and aiming) in boys and found incremental improvements until puberty, when skills reached a plateau. The development of motor skills is not necessarily related to physical maturity, as children who become stronger, taller, and heavier with age may not similarly increase their levels of motor skill development.[3]

Seefeldt,[4] who evaluated eight fundamental motor skills to determine when children would be able to perform specific tasks, discovered the age at which 60% of boys and girls could perform each of the following tasks: throwing, kicking, running, jumping, catching, striking, hopping, and skipping. The evidence indicates that the preschool child can perform some of these tasks; by early elementary school, the child can do most of them. Then, the child can learn to refine these motor skills through repetitive practice.

Almost all the children followed the same sequence in progressing from the rudimentary to the mature stages of performance. This was true whether the child was normal or handicapped by a developmental disability or blindness. Since blind children could not watch others perform these tasks, there must be an ingrained progression of motor skill acquisition.

Physical educators have demonstrated through cross-sectional studies that efficiency of movement improves during childhood and adolescence. The major longitudinal study was that of Branta and associates,[1] who studied children 5 through 10 years old and 8 through 14 years old. Semiannual measurements were taken of the flexed-arm hang, jump and reach, 120-foot agility run, standing long jump, 30-yard dash, sit and reach, and 400-foot shuttle run. Although boys exhibited greater stability in performing the motor tasks than did girls, there was a surprising amount of instability, particularly with younger children and in certain tests.

There is little evidence to indicate that one can predict a child's readiness to learn specific motor skills on the basis of chronological age, body size, or other assessments of biologic maturation. Sport-specific tests of certain motor skills may be able to predict success in that sport, but not sports readiness. The tests involve a task analysis of the skills to be learned, and selection of the most important skills that can be used for prediction. Studies of young hockey players have identified the most proficient players.[5,6]

Conclusion

Medical practitioners must rely on their common sense when assessing sports readiness. A permissive answer, based on the child's eagerness to try, is better than preventing participation because of a vague feeling that the child is "too young" or "immature."

References

1. Branta C, Haubenstricker J, Seefeldt V: Age changes in motor skills during childhood and adolescence. *Exerc Sport Sci Rev* 1984;12:467-520.
2. Bodie DA: Changes in lung function, ballhandling skills, and performance measures during adolescence in normal school boys, in Binkhorst RA, et al (eds): *Children and Exercise XI*. Champaign, Human Kinetics, 1985, pp 260-268.
3. Kemper HCG, Verschuur R: Motor performance fitness tests, in Kemper HCG (ed): *Growth, Health, and Physical Fitness of Teenagers*. Basel, 1985, vol 20, pp 96-106.
4. Seefeldt V: The concept of readiness applied to motor skills acquisition, in Magill RA, Ash MJ, Smoll FL (eds): *Children in Sport*, ed 2. Champaign, Human Kinetics, 1982, pp 31-37.
5. MacNab RB: A longitudinal study of ice hockey in boys aged 8-12. *Can J Appl Sport Sci* 1979;4:11-17.
6. Hermiston RT, Gratto J, Teno T: Three hockey skills tests as predictors of hockey playing ability. *Can J Appl Sport Sci* 1979;4:95-97.

Consensus Statements: Training

1. Although children are equal to adults in aerobic capacity, children have a higher metabolic cost for endurance activities.
2. Improvements in aerobic capacity are related more to periods of rapid growth than to the effects of training.
3. Children have reduced anaerobic capacity compared with adults.
4. Children can make the same muscle strength gains as adults in response to properly supervised training programs.
5. There is no scientific information to determine the psychologic and physical risks to children from systematic aerobic and anaerobic overload. More information is needed.
6. There are eight fundamental motor skills used in sport: throwing, kicking, running, jumping, catching, striking, hopping, and skipping. However, sport-specific tests are not sufficient to determine a child's sport readiness.
7. Clinicians must rely on common sense to determine the sport readiness of a child and concentrate on the child's eagerness to participate.
8. Strenuous training is less effective before the growth spurt than after it and may lead to early "burn out."
9. Coaches who work with young athletes need specific information about training techniques. Educational programs in this area should be required.

Section Two

Nutrition and Drugs

Chapter 6

Vitamins and Supplements

Michael Nelson, MD

Athletes have used and abused nutritional compounds since the inception of athletic competition. Throughout history, a wide range of foods and nutritional products have been used to enhance performance. Currently, there is a great deal of interest in the use of calcium, iron, and protein. This chapter focuses on the use of these supplements.

Calcium

Calcium is the major component of bone mineral. In soft tissue, it plays an important role in cellular metabolism, including mitochondrial functioning, the formation of cyclic adenosine monophosphate, and the modulation of excitatory thresholds.[1]

The amount of calcium needed to sustain bone mineral integrity varies with age, stage of development, and growth rate. There is no evidence to indicate that exercise increases these requirements.

Recommendations for daily intake vary among organizations. (Table 1.) In the United States, the National Academy of Sciences recommends 800 mg/day for children and 1,200 mg/day for adolescents. The World Health Organization recommendations are considerably lower—400 to 500 mg/day for children and 600 to 700 mg/day for adolescents.[2]

Dietary calcium is especially important for women. Low calcium intake may contribute to osteoporosis in amenorrheic athletes. Although the causes of amenorrhea and osteoporosis are not clear, most studies have shown that excessive exercise, hypoestrogenemia, and poor diet are contributory.[3]

Some female athletes, particularly gymnasts and ballet dancers, have notoriously poor diets, which frequently contain less than the recommended intake of calcium and other nutrients. How the low calcium intake contributes to osteoporosis in relation to the athlete's hypoestrogenemic state and the intensity of exercise is not entirely clear.

Athletes whose calcium intake is below recommended guidelines should include a supplement in their diet. The best supplement is a change in diet to increase intake of dairy products, fish, almonds, broc-

Table 1. Recommended Daily Supplements of Vitamins and Minerals

Supplement	Children	Adolescents
Calcium	800 mg*	1200 mg*
	400 mg**	700 mg**
Iron	18 mg***	65-day supplement
	(available in a 3000-calorie	3 mg/kg replacement
	diet)	
Protein	1.2–1.5 gm***	
Vitamins, Minerals	supplement unnecessary for either children or	
	adolescents***	

* National Academy of Sciences
** World Health Organization
*** Available in daily diet

coli, or navy and soy beans. Any calcium carbonate over-the-counter supplement is also acceptable. Calcium carbonate contains 40% calcium (for example, an antacid with 500 mg of calcium carbonate has 200 mg of calcium).[1-3]

In the amenorrheic athlete, an evaluation of the athlete's estrogen status and a search for the cause of the amenorrhea (including a pregnancy test) should be done before prescribing a calcium supplement. In selected athletes an estrogen supplement and/or a reduction in the intensity of exercise may be needed in addition to a calcium supplement.

Iron

Iron deficiency is the most common nutritional deficit in the United States. Iron is essential for the formation of hemoglobin, myoglobin, and some enzymes, and for the metabolic function of cytochromes.[4]

Iron deficiency (less than 12 g/dl of serum ferritin) has been reported in 20% to 24% of adolescent females and 12% of adolescent males. Most studies show an increased incidence of either iron deficiency or associated anemia in athletes.[5] One study of teenage cross-country runners revealed an incidence of iron deficiency in 17% of males and in 45% of females,[6] using a serum ferritin level of 18 g/dl as a lower limit of normal. Since many of these athletes did not become deficient until well into the running season, their iron deficiency would have been missed without periodic testing during the season. The increased occurrence of iron deficiency may result from iron losses through sweat, feces, urine, or hemolysis.

Although significant anemia (hemoglobin level of less than 11 g/dl) has a negative effect on exercise performance, the impact of iron deficiency is less clear. Some researchers[4,7] have shown that treating previously iron-deficient athletes improves endurance and Vo_2 max and reduces muscle lactate. Others have not found that iron supplements improve performance or fitness in nonanemic iron-deficient subjects. However, more evidence indicates that iron supplements are beneficial to the deficient athlete.

Screening all athletes for iron deficiency (increased anemia) is not currently cost-effective. The physician may provide iron supplements on the basis of selective screening for risk factors such as inadequate dietary intake, hypermenorrhea, or the presence of chronic disease. Or, the physician may recommend iron supplements for all athletes without screening. Both of these alternatives have drawbacks. Perhaps an inexpensive way to screen all athletes will be developed in the near future.

The US National Academy of Science currently recommends 18 mg/day of elemental iron for adolescents. A 3,000-calorie intake is needed to provide this amount of iron with the typical American diet.

A recommended dose of 65 mg/day of elemental iron, in addition to a regular diet, may protect athletes from iron deficiency. This dosage (in excess of the recommended daily allowance) allows for fecal wastage. However, in previous studies many iron-deficient athletes were already taking an iron supplement when they were tested.

If the physician suspects iron deficiency, a serum ferritin level should be obtained. The recommendation for iron replacement is 3 mg/kg/day.[2] Foods high in iron include red meat, poultry, fish, whole grain or enriched breads, and cereals. Many available over-the-counter iron supplements are acceptable alternatives.

Protein

Recently studies have shown that athletes may need more protein in their diets than the recommended daily allowance.[8,9] The evidence is not conclusive because of variations in energy intake, energy expenditure, methods of determining protein utilization, and duration of the studies.

In the short term, protein catabolism and amino acid oxidation increase during and after exercise. After a period of adaptation to exercise, the athlete's need for increased protein may diminish or disappear completely.[10,11]

Protein need varies with energy intake. If the diet does not meet the body's energy needs for exercise activity, protein need can increase dramatically because of the breakdown of lean body mass.

Protein requirements vary directly with energy expenditure. Increasing intensity from 40% to 50% Vo_2 max to 64% Vo_2 max can more than double the protein required to maintain nitrogen balance.

Regardless of these research limitations, the protein requirements of athletes may be as much as 20% to 50% higher than the requirements of nonathletes. Adolescents in general need an estimated 1 gram of protein per kilogram of body weight daily. Even if the adolescent athlete needs 1.2 to 1.5 g/kg/day, the diet of the typical American teenager provides far more protein. Using protein supplements in addition to the average diet is expensive, unnecessary, and potentially harmful to the athlete because they may increase the acid load on the renal system. They may also decrease endurance.

Although there may be other nutritional deficits in an adolescent athlete's diet, there is no evidence to support the concept that taking vitamin or mineral supplements in addition to a normal diet will enhance performance. Too much of these substrates may be harmful. If an athlete's diet supplies less than 70% of the recommended daily allowances, it can be supplemented with a multiple vitamin.[1]

References

1. Berning JR: Nutritional demands of the growing athlete, in *Proceedings of the American College of Sports Medicine Clinical Conference*. Indianapolis, American College of Sports Medicine, 1988.

2. American Academy of Pediatrics, Committee on Nutrition: *Pediatric Nutrition Handbook*, ed 2. Elk Grove Village, Illinois, American Academy of Pediatrics, 1985.

3. American Academy of Pediatrics, Committee on Sports Medicine: Amenorrhea in adolescent athletes. *Pediatrics*, in press.

4. Belko AZ: Vitamins and exercise: An update. *Med Sci Sports Exerc* 1987; 19:S191-S196.

5. Rowland TW, Block SA, Kelleher JF: Iron deficiency in adolescent endurance athetes. *J Adoles Health Care* 1987;8:322-326.

6. Risser WL, Lee EJ, et al: Iron deficiency in female athletes: Its prevalence and impact on performance. *Med Sci Sports Exerc* 1988;20:116-121.

7. Rowland TW, Deisroth MD, et al: The effect of iron therapy on the exercise capacity of nonanemic iron-deficient adolescent runners. *Am J Dis Child* 1988;142:165-169.

8. Lemon WR: Protein and exercise: Update 1987. *Ned Sci Sports Exerc* 1987; 19:S179-S190.

9. Lemon WR: Protein utilization, letter. *Med Sci Sports Exerc* 1988;20:416-417.

10. Butterfield GE: Whole body protein utilization in humans. *Med Sci Sports Exerc* 1987;19:S157-S165.

11. Butterfield GE: Protein utilization, letter. *Med Sci Sports Exerc* 1988;20:415-416.

Chapter 7

Fluid and Electrolyte Issues

Jerry Vannatta, MD

This discussion includes only those electrolytes currently known to be clinically relevant, although others may prove to be so in the future.

Normal Salt and Water Balance

Total body water, which makes up 60% of body weight, is divisible into three parts: (1) the plasma (intravascular) and (2) interstitial compartments, which together constitute the extracellular fluid space, and (3) the intracellular fluid space. The electrolyte content of the compartments (Table 1) can only be estimated and will vary from person to person.

In this discussion pediatric data are used whenever possible. However, in some areas no data exist for this age group and research from older subjects is substituted. This is an important point because the ratio of body mass to surface area differs significantly in prepubertal and postpubertal athletes. Postpubertal athletes appear to have adult body mass to surface area ratios. This allows one to deal with them as adults with regard to water and electrolytes.

Sodium and Potassium Concentrations in Sweat

Water and electrolyte loss via sweating becomes clinically significant as the volume of sweat increases. To estimate electrolyte losses in an exercising athlete, the electrolyte content of sweat must be known.

Interestingly, published articles disagree because the concentrations of sodium (Na^+) and potassium (K^+) are apparently affected by the rate of sweating, the age of the athlete, and the technique used for the measurement.

Sodium Content The concentration of Na^+ in sweat varies with sweat volume in a linear fashion, so that as flow increases, Na^+ concentration increases. Schwartz and Thaysen[1] showed that after injection of B-methylacetylcholine into the forearms of adults the concentration of Na^+ var-

Table 1. Electrolyte Content of Body Water Compartments

Ion	Compartment	mEq/L
Na^+	Plasma; interstitial fluid	140
K^+	Plasma; interstitial fluid	4
	Intracellular fluid	150
$PO_4^=$	Intracellular fluid	97
Cl^-	Plasma; interstitial fluid	103
$SO_4^=$	Intracellular fluid	20
HCO_3^-	Plasma; interstitial fluid	27
Mg^{2+}	Plasma; interstitial fluid	3
	Intracellular fluid	45
Ca^{2+}	Plasma; interstitial fluid	5

ied from 1.9 to 103 mEq/L. They also found that K^+ concentrations ranged from 5 to 28 mEq/L, with an average of 9.4 mEq/L.

Lobeck and Huebner[2] performed sweat analyses on children and adults and reported similar results. When sweating was induced by pilocarpine ionophoresis, the K^+ concentration was age-, sex-, and flow-independent, and averaged 9 to 10 mEq/L. However, Costill and associates[3] and Dill and associates,[4] using the body washdown method, reported K^+ concentrations averaging 4.5 to 5.0 mEq/L. The only apparent explanation for this discrepancy is that the higher K^+ values were found in nonconditioned subjects with sweating induced by cholinergic drugs whereas the lower values were in moderately to well-conditioned athletes with sweating induced by exercise in a heated environment.

Shifts of Water and Solute With Exercise

Exercise shifts water and electrolytes from and between the plasma and the interstitial compartments and the extracellular and intracellular fluid spaces. With short bursts of exercise, hypotonic fluid (water) shifts from the plasma to the intracellular compartment. This was originally demonstrated by Jacobsson and Kjellmer.[5] Other investigators[6] have shown that this shift occurs in three phases. At rest the interstitial, vascular, and intracellular spaces are in their normal state. At the end of a one-minute burst of full-intensity fatiguing exercise (phase 1), the plasma volume decreases by approximately 10% and the serum sodium concentration increases. Thus, solute-free water enters the cellular compartment, leaving the extracellular compartment contracted and hypertonic. During the first four minutes of recovery (phase 2), water is thought to enter the interstitial space, followed by sodium from the vascular space. Finally, over the next 60 minutes (phase 3), isotonic fluid is recaptured from the interstitial space to reexpand the vascular volume.

This is very unlike all other known states of hypernatremia, which are associated with significant water deficits. Serum sodium concentrations are unlikely to be noticed by a physician within four or five minutes of exercise, but it is important to be aware of this phenomenon.

Costill and associates,[7] who studied adult men exercising in a heated environment, measured electrolyte and water losses and shifts. During approximately 90 minutes of continuous exercise the subjects lost 2.2%, 4.1%, and 5.8% of their normal body weights as a result of dehydration; approximately two-thirds of the water lost was from the extracellular space and one-third was from the intracellular space.

In these experiments, by the time the subjects had lost 5.8% of their body weights, they had lost approximately 10 mEq of K^+ and 160 mEq of Na^+. The urine contained approximately 8 mEq/L of sodium and 7 mEq/L of potassium, representing approximately 6.3% of total body sodium and 8.7% of total body potassium. Nonetheless, the ratio of extracellular to intracellular potassium (Ke/Ki) did not change and consequently neither did membrane potentials, probably because significant amounts of interstitial K^+ moved into both fluid compartments.

This exercise study took approximately 90 minutes. Thus, during a relatively short exercise session in a heated environment, the loss of approximately 45 mEq of potassium is apparently compensated for by replacement from the interstitial space, and intracellular potassium is not significantly disturbed.

Water Requirements   Several studies have suggested that children sweat less than adults do when exercising in a heated environment.[8,9] They have also been shown to voluntarily hypohydrate under such conditions. Bar-Or and associates[10] compared two groups of 10- to 12-year-old boys. One group voluntarily hydrated (children were allowed free access to water) during a 3.5-hour exercise session and the second group was force-hydrated (children were instructed to ingest water at a predetermined rate). The first group suffered a statistically significant greater weight loss and had less fluid intake. This group had higher rectal temperatures and showed greater heat stress. In fact, the heat stress in this group of children was similar to that in obese adults and much greater than that seen in lean adults.

There seem to be several reasons for this inability of children to respond as well as adults to exercise in the heat. (1) Children have a greater ratio of surface area to body mass. This becomes a deterrent when ambient temperature is greater than skin temperature. (2) Tasks such as walking and running are metabolically more expensive to children than to young adults. (3) As a group, 10- to 12-year-old boys have greater adiposity than adolescents or young adults. This is a handicap in the heat. (4) Cardiac output at a given metabolic rate is somewhat lower in children than in adults. This might limit convection of heat from core to periphery. (5) Children sweat less than adults while performing similar tasks in hot environments.

Water requirements may be higher in children than in adults, and children must be made to drink more than they would ingest voluntarily to avoid heat stress if they exercise for long periods in a hot environment.

Dress During Exercise   The type of clothing worn during exercise in a hot environment affects the body's ability to utilize evaporative cooling. In the study by Mathews and associates,[11] young men exercising on a treadmill wore either a full football uniform, or a pair of shorts and no shirt. Those dressed in shorts wore backpacks weighing the same as the football uniforms. The athletes wearing uniforms had much higher rectal temperatures because the uniforms permitted only 30% to 40% of the sweat to be evaporated whereas the shorts and packs permitted approximately 70% to be evaporated. Thus, in addition to heat and humidity, dress is an important factor in determining how much heat stress a given amount of exercise produces and, therefore, the water requirements of the athlete.

Sex Differences   The sexes differ in their response to exercise in a heated environment. Dill and associates[4] studied 14 male and 12 female high-school athletes who performed aerobic exercise in 40 C heat. Sweat rates and volumes were higher for males than females but final rectal temperatures were not different. There were also no differences in the sodium and chloride contents of the sweat. Therefore, although boys lose more sweat volume than girls, girls appear to be at no disadvantage in regard to temperature regulation.

Percentage of Body Fat   Haymes and associates[9] studied lean and obese prepubertal boys and their sweating response to exercise. They defined lean as less than 20% body fat and obese as more than 24% body fat. The boys walked on a treadmill for three 20-minute exercise periods at various temperatures. Total sweat rates were equal, but heat production, measured by rectal temperatures, was higher in obese boys.

Electrolyte Shifts and Losses With Exercise

Sodium   It has been shown that exercise has an effect on the renal handling of Na^+. Costill and associates[3] showed that 60 minutes of exercise in adults significantly increases plasma renin activity and serum aldosterone concentrations. The urine Na^+ concentration decreases during the exercise period and plasma volume expands. The expanded plasma volume is the result of increased fractional reabsorption of sodium and water.

Simultaneously, the athlete loses fairly large volumes of sweat. Na^+ concentration and volume vary, depending on sex, age, percent of body fat, ambient temperature, and dress. However, if the Na^+ concentration is estimated to be 30 mEq/L/day and the volume is estimated to be 6/L/day, the athlete might lose 180 mEq of Na^+ during a 60-minute workout.

This raises the question of replacement with water containing electrolytes. In a cross-over study of 12 adult athletes participating in two five-day experimental sessions separated by three control days, one group had their sweat losses replaced with electrolyte-free water and a second group had their losses replaced with an electrolyte-containing solution. The subjects in the first group accumulated more Na^+. This seemingly paradoxical finding is explained by the fact that the subjects who received the electrolyte solution had higher urine volumes with higher Na^+ contents. It appears that the intake of fluid containing Na^+ during the exercise period decreased aldosterone secretion, thereby increasing Na^+ in the urine.

The average daily intake of sodium in the American diet is approximately 200 mEq. Even if 6 L of water is lost, the sodium balance remains positive (200 mEq ingested and 180 mEq lost). Therefore, if the athlete's diet contains an average amount of sodium, supplementation is not needed.

Potassium Knochel and associates[12] studied a group of young men in basic training. These experiments were conducted under conditions similar to those used in athletic training and the results were applicable to postpubertal athletes. During the 32-day training period, training in a heated environment produced a loss of 345 mEq of K^+ despite adequate potassium intake (100 mEq/day). Serum potassium concentrations, however, did not fall below normal. They also noted that trainees who exercised in a heated environment had blunted aldosterone responses when compared with those who exercised in cool weather. This occurred when there was a K^+ deficit in the sweat but the serum K^+ concentration was normal.

It has been shown that K^+ shifts from the intracellular space to plasma during both short-term and long-term aerobic exercise. The plasma increase is usually between 0.5 and 1.0/mEq/L.[13,14]

Costill and associates[15] studied the effects of two different low-K^+ diets on adults and their responses to exercise. One diet contained 8 mEq/day and the other 25 mEq/day. Each diet lasted four days, during which time the subjects exercised. They found a net gain of K^+, even with the low-potassium diet, and concluded that no dietary supplement is needed.

These findings are difficult to interpret. The two studies used different methods and the estimated concentration of K^+ in sweat was 4.5 mEq/L in one[15] and 9.0 mEq/L in the other.[12] Knochel and associates[12] concluded that K^+ deficits occur with exercise in a heated environment and Costill and associates[15] concluded that they do not.

Since serum K^+ is increased by both aerobic and anaerobic exercise, it seems judicious to avoid K^+ supplementation during or shortly after exercise. Both studies support the suggestion that a diet containing 100 mEq/day of K^+ would avoid serious hypokalemia and K^+ deficit in the athlete.

A problem might arise in an athlete whose diet is low in potassium and who exercises in a heated environment for two or three weeks. Costill and associates[15] measured the K^+ balance only during a four-day period.

For example, if a large, postpubertal athlete participates in two exercise sessions per day in the summer heat, preparing for football, and he eats doughnuts for breakfast and a hamburger and french fries for lunch and dinner, with each meal accompanied by a soft drink, his diet would contain approximately 50 mEq/L of potassium. Assuming a 6-L water loss per day, and a sweat K^+ concentration of 5 mEq/L, this athlete would lose 30 mEq/day. Urine K^+ losses would average 30 to 40 mEq/day, producing a K^+ deficit. If the sweat K^+ concentration was 10 mEq/L, the deficit would be greater. On the other hand, if this same athlete ate a normal, well-balanced diet containing 100 mEq/day, there would be no deficit.

Disorders Associated With Electrolyte and Water Loss

Heat Cramps   This manifestation of heat stress is thought to be secondary to sodium depletion although good evidence is lacking. The condition is readily identified by muscle cramping and easily treated with copious amounts of water and additional sodium ingestion.

Heat Exhaustion   This usually represents failure of the heat-regulating mechanisms brought on by high temperatures. Sweating ceases, the skin becomes dry and hot, and the body temperature rises to dangerous levels.

Prepubertal athletes are at greater risk for heat stress than postpubertal athletes and adults. Children with the following conditions are at even greater risk: obesity, febrile state, cystic fibrosis, gastrointestinal infection, diabetes insipidus, diabetes mellitus, chronic heart failure, caloric malnutrition, anorexia nervosa, sweating insufficiency, and mental deficiency.[16]

Avoiding heat stroke requires acclimatizing the athlete to exercise in the heat. It is an important factor in early-season workouts and in athletes who have moved from a cool dry climate to a hot and/or damp climate.

Acclimatization data were collected by Wagner and associates.[17] In their study, prepubertal boys, 11 to 14 years old, were compared with older pubescent boys, 15 to 16 years old. Although ratio of body surface area to mass was greater in the younger boys, they were less efficient at temperature regulation because they had less ability to sweat.

This study also suggested that eight days may be a reasonable acclimatization time for older boys, but not long enough for prepubertal boys to regulate their body temperatures well.

Summary

The following guidelines can be used to avoid water and electrolyte depletion:

Early in the season, when athletes are poorly conditioned, workouts should be less strenuous and water breaks frequent.

Prepubertal athletes are at increased risk for heat exhaustion and heat cramps. Obese children and children with other diseases are more susceptible to dehydration, heat exhaustion, and heat cramps.

Because the volume of sweat varies greatly from person to person, athletes should be weighed before and after practice, to allow an estimate of total water loss. Since most athletes tend to become hypohydrated, a water prescription may be needed.

Total sodium loss also varies but, within physiologic limits, a well-balanced diet should replace all sodium lost in the sweat. Salt substitutes should not be needed, and should be avoided. A well-balanced diet should replace potassium lost in the sweat, and supplements should not be needed. Potassium supplements should be avoided during competition and shortly thereafter.

Water should be replaced during competition with an electrolyte-free solution. This avoids unnecessarily high urine volumes during competition.

References

1. Schwartz IL, Thaysen JH: Excretion of sodium and potassium in human sweat. *J Clin Invest* 1956;35:114-120.
2. Lobeck CC, Huebner D: Effect of age, sex, and cystic fibrosis on the sodium and potassium content of human sweat. *Pediatrics* 1962;30:172-179.
3. Costill DL, Coté R, Miller E, et al: Water and electrolyte replacement during repeated days of work in the heat. *Aviat Space Environ Med* 1975;46:795-800.
4. Dill DB, Soholt LF, McLean DC, et al: Capacity of young males and females for running in desert heat. *Med Sci Sports* 1977;9:137-142.
5. Jacobsson S, Kjellmer I: Flow and protein content of lymph in resting and exercising skeletal muscle. *Acta Physiol Scand* 1964;60:278-285.
6. Sejersted OM, Vøllestad NK, Medbø JI: Muscle fluid and electrolyte balance during and following exercise. *Acta Physiol Scand* 1986;128(suppl 556):119-127.
7. Costill DL, Coté R, Fink W: Muscle water and electrolytes following varied levels of dehydration in man. *J Appl Physiol* 1976;40:6-11.
8. Drinkwater BL, Kupprat IC, Denton JE, et al: Response of prepubertal girls and college women to work in the heat. *J Appl Physiol* 1977;43:1046-1053.
9. Haymes EM, McCormick RJ, Buskirk ER: Heat tolerance of exercising lean and obese prepubertal boys. *J Appl Physiol* 1975;39:457-461.
10. Bar-Or O, Dotan R, Inbar O, et al: Voluntary hypohydration in 10-to 12-year-old boys. *J Appl Physiol* 1980;48:104-108.
11. Mathews DK, Fox EL, Tamzo D: Physiological responses during exercise and recovery in a football uniform. *J Appl Physiol* 1969;26:611-615.
12. Knochel P, Dotin LN, Hamburger RJ: Pathophysiology of intense physical conditioning in a hot climate: I. Mechanisms of potassium depletion. *J Clin Invest* 1972;51:242-255.
13. William ME, Gervino EV, Rosa RM, et al: Catecholamine modulation of rapid potassium shifts during exercise. *N Engl J Med* 1985;312:823-827.
14. Rose LI, Carroll DR, Lowe SL, et al: Serum electrolyte changes after marathon running. *J Appl Physiol* 1970;29:449-451.
15. Costill DL, Coté R, Fink WJ: Dietary potassium and heavy exercise: Effects on muscle water and electrolytes. *Am J Clin Nutr* 1982;36:266-275.
16. Committee on Sports Medicine, American Academy of Pediatrics: Climatic heat stress and the exercising child. *Pediatrics* 1982;69:808-809.
17. Wagner JA, Robinson S, Tzankoff SP, et al: Heat tolerance and acclimatization to work in the heat in relation to age. *J Appl Physiol* 1972;33:616-622.

Chapter 8

Drugs and Ergogenic Aids

John A. Lombardo, MD

Drug use among athletes is always a difficult topic to discuss. Often the discussion encompasses marijuana, caffeine, cortisone, cocaine, and anabolic steroids with no acknowledgment that these drugs vary widely in their effects. Drugs used by athletes can be divided into three categories: therapeutic, performance-enhancing, and "recreational drugs" used for entertainment or escape. This chapter focuses on performance-enhancing agents.

Prevalence of Use

Although performance-enhancing drugs and ergogenic aids have only recently received widespread publicity, athletes have been trying ever since competition began to improve their performances through the use of high-intensity and advanced-training techniques, improved diets, and various performance-enhancing agents such as the hearts of bulls and courageous opponents, special concoctions, herbs, and drugs. The use of performance-enhancing agents creates a "trickle-down" effect. Young fans model themselves after their heroes, using the same techniques and equipment, even wearing the same hairstyle. Advertisers take advantage of this adulation by employing heroes to market products.

To what extent professional, college, and elite amateur athletes use performance-enhancing agents is not known because of the negative public image connected with their use. Users are afraid of being identified, so it is difficult to assess the accuracy of survey results, even when the surveys are anonymous. This leads to a great deal of speculation, some educated and some ill-founded. The only accurate conclusions that can be drawn from these surveys are that performance-enhancing agents are used, and that they are used at all levels (high school through professional).[1-3]

Performance-Enhancing Agents

Performance-enhancing agents can be divided into three types: anabolic agents, stimulants, and relaxants.

For each type of agent, the following questions can be asked: How does the drug work? Why do athletes use it? What are the known adverse effects?

Anabolic Agents Anabolic agents enhance performance by increasing lean body mass, increasing strength, and enabling the athlete to perform frequent high-intensity workouts. Anabolic-androgenic steroids, growth hormone, and amino acids are three anabolic agents used by athletes.

Anabolic-Androgenic Steroids These analogs of the male hormone testosterone have both androgenic (masculinizing) effects and anabolic (tissue-building) effects. They are used by athletes in a short-acting oral form and a long-acting injectable form. Their intended medical use is as a testosterone replacement.

The medical and scientific communities denied the effectiveness of anabolic-androgenic steroids for many years.[4,5] A critical evaluation of the literature does show that anabolic-androgenic steroids effectively increase lean body mass and strength when used in combination with high-intensity workouts and a proper diet.[6] Athletes report that these drugs allow them to perform frequent high-intensity workouts without breaking down. Consequently, the users include athletes who perform frequent high-intensity work (runners and swimmers) as well as strength athletes (lifters, football players, throwers).

Anabolic-androgenic steroids have many adverse effects.[6] Psychologically, they may cause increased aggressiveness, mood swings, and libidinal changes. Adverse physical effects include changes in the liver (cholestasis and metabolic changes, benign or malignant tumors, and peliosis hepatitis), the cardiovascular system (increased blood pressure and decreased high-density lipoprotein cholesterol [HDL-C]), the immune system (increased natural killer-cell activity and decreased immunoglobulin A [IgA] and immunoglobulin M [IgM]), and the musculoskeletal system (weakened connective tissues). In men, anabolic-androgenic steroids can lead to oligospermia or azoospermia, testicular atrophy, prostatic hypertrophy, and testicular or prostatic tumors. In women, irreversible masculinization (clitoral enlargement, changes in hair patterns, deepening of the voice) and menstrual changes may occur. The young or skeletally immature athlete runs the risk of premature closure of growth plates or early maturation. Other adverse effects may be irreversible alopecia, acne, or irreversible gynecomastia.

Most of these effects are temporary and reverse when the drugs are removed. Some adverse effects may be related to duration, dose, and frequency of the drug, while others occur regardless of these factors.

Growth Hormone Growth hormone or somatotropin is a polypeptide hormone produced by the anterior pituitary gland. Growth hormone is attractive to athletes because it increases protein anabolism, enhances tissue repair, and increases fat metabolism.[7]

There are no studies on the effects of growth hormone on the athlete. Even anecdotal reports by athletes are not as reliable as those for anabolic steroids.

The adverse effects of growth hormone are the same as those found in acromegaly. They include bone changes (coarsening and deformity) in the hands, feet, skull, and face; soft-tissue thickening; glucose intolerance; hypertension; atherosclerosis; cardiomyopathy, and myopathy.[8]

With the development of the DNA-recombinant method of production, growth hormone will become more available and its abuse may increase among athletes.

Amino Acids   Amino acids stimulate the release of growth hormone. Lysine, arginine, and ornithine are the most popular. Lysine and arginine can be taken orally to stimulate growth hormone release.[9] There are no studies concerning the effectiveness of amino acids nor are there any reports of adverse effects.

Stimulants   The popularity of stimulants has diminished since the days of Mandell's "Sunday syndrome."[10] Stimulants can increase energy, decrease fat, increase aggressiveness, and enhance performance. The two most frequently used stimulants are amphetamines and caffeine.

Amphetamines   Amphetamines are indirect-acting sympathomimetic agents. Their effectiveness is questionable. Some studies laud their effectiveness[11-14] whereas others refute the claimed positive effects.[15,16] Adverse effects include ventricular arrhythmia, insomnia, tremors, anxiety, toxic psychosis, and confusion.[17]

Caffeine   Caffeine is found in some colas, tea, coffee, and chocolate. It is used by athletes because it has a stimulating effect on the central nervous system and may provide a metabolic advantage as well.[17]

It is difficult to compare the numerous studies on the metabolic effects of caffeine in the athlete. This difficulty results from the lack of uniformity in study design and the small numbers of athletes studied. However, an attempt to summarize the available data is worthwhile.

There are two hypotheses regarding the metabolic advantage of caffeine ingestion in athletes. The first is that caffeine causes increased lipolysis, thus releasing free fatty acids into the blood and making them available as metabolic substrate. This could conceivably lead to carbohydrate-sparing and enhanced performance. The second hypothsis is that caffeine affects glycogen mobilization by inhibiting glycogen phosphorylase.

Attempts to test these hypotheses have provided conflicting results. Some studies sustained the glycogen-sparing effects of caffeine but others did not. The effects of caffeine on the free fatty acids and on gylcogen-sparing may depend on the subject's long-term caffeine ingestion. Thus, if the subject regularly ingests caffeine, an injection of caffeine will not cause a significant increase in free fatty acids. On the other hand, if the subject is caffeine-deprived before the experiment, there may be a significant increase in free fatty acids, and some studies have shown enhanced performance under these circumstances. These data would be consistent with a metabolic tolerance of the drug.[18]

Another variable is the nutritional state of the subject before ingesting caffeine. Some studies suggest that a high-carbohydrate diet

(70% of total calories) for three days before exercise and a high-carbohydrate meal taken with the caffeine negate the expected increase in free fatty acids, and the carbohydrate-sparing effects.[19]

A reasonable statement is that caffeine, when taken under the correct set of circumstances, may enhance endurance performance. At this time, however, the correct set of circumstances is not known.

Ingesting caffeine can have some adverse effects, including cardiac arrhythmias tremors, insomnia, and diuresis.

Relaxants   Relaxation is desirable in activities that stress fine skills, such as figure skating, archery, and shooting. Participants have used propranolol, a beta-blocker, as an aid to relaxation.[20]

Ethical and Legal Issues

Should the use of drugs as ergogenic aids be allowed in sports? Should the decision to use drugs depend on the individual's freedom of choice in weighing risks and benefits? At the present time, many governing bodies (including the IOC, the USOC, and the NCAA) forbid the use of drugs to enhance performance. The role of performance-enhancing agents at any level is questionable, and they certainly have no place among pediatric athletes.

Nonetheless, the belief that "winning is everything; therefore, win at all costs" can be used to rationalize and justify the use of drugs to enhance performance. The team physician is responsible for the health and safety of the athlete. In keeping with this role, the medical community should continue to educate athletes, coaches, and parents, to perform research and detection testing, and to strive for a philosophical view that performance-enhancing drug use is not justifiable.

References

1. Clement DB: Drug use survey: Results and conclusions. *Phys Sportsmed* 1983;11:64-67.
2. Ljungqvist A: The use of anabolic steroids in top Swedish athletes. *Br J Sports Med* 1975;9:82.
3. Anderson WA, McKeag DB: The substance use and abuse of college-student athletes. *Sport Doc*, 1986, vol 22.
4. American College of Sports Medicine: Position statement on the use and abuse of anabolic/androgenic steroids in sports. *Med Sci Sports* 1977;9:xi-xiii.
5. Ryan AJ: Anabolic steroids are fool's gold. *Fed Proc* 1981;40:2682-2688.
6. American College of Sports Medicine: Position stand on the use of anabolic/androgenic steroids in sports. *Med Sci Sports* 1984;19:xiii-xviii.
7. Macintyre JG: Growth hormone and athletes. *Sports Med* 1987;4:129-142.
8. Linfoot JA: Acromegaly and giantism, in Daugheday (ed): *Endocrine Control of Growth*. New York, Elsevier, 1981.
9. Isidori A, Lo Monaco A, Cappa M: A study of growth hormone release in man after oral administration of amino acids. *Curr Med Res Opin* 1981;7:475-481.
10. Mandell AJ: The Sunday syndrome: A unique pattern of amphetamine abuse indigenous to American professional football. *Clin Toxicol* 1979;15:225-232.

11. Smith GM, Beecher HK: Amphetamine sulfate and athletic performance. *JAMA* 1959;170:542-557.

12. Smith GM, Beecher HK: Amphetamine, secobarbital, and athletic performance: II. Subjective evaluation of performances, mood states and physical state. *JAMA* 1960;172:1502-1514.

13. Smith GM, Weitzner M, Beecher HK: Increased sensitivity of measurement of drug effects in expert swimmers. *J Pharmacol Exp Ther* 1963;139:114-119.

14. Chandler JV, Blair SN: The effect of amphetamines on selected physiological components related to athletic success. *Med Sci Sports Exerc* 1980;12:65-69.

15. Karpovich PV: Effect of amphetamine sulfate on athletic performance. *JAMA* 1950;170:558-561.

16. Golding L, Barnarda JR: The effect of *d*-amphetamine sulfate on physical performance. *J Sports Med* 1963;3:221-224.

17. Lombardao JA: Stimulants, in Strauss RH (ed): *Drugs and Performance in Sports*. Philadelphia, WB Saunders, 1987, pp 69-85.

18. Fisher SM, McMurray RG, Berry M, et al: Influence of caffeine on exercise performance in habitual caffeine users. *Int J Sports Med* 1986;7:276-280.

19. Weir J, Noakes TD, Myburgh K, et al: A high carbohydrate diet negates the metabolic effects of caffeine during erercise. *Med Sci Sports Exerc* 1987;19:100-105.

20. Lombardo JA: Depressants, in Strauss RH (ed): *Drugs and Performance in Sports*. Philadelphia, WB Saunders, 1987, pp 87-102.

Medical Care for the Pediatric Athlete

Chapter 9

Preparticipation Evaluation

John A. Lombardo, MD

Every athlete has the right to a "thorough preseason history and medical evaluation," according to the American Medical Association Committee on Medical Aspects of Sports.[1] As sports medicine developed, the preparticipation evaluation progressed from a "locker-room lineup" to a sophisticated physical examination and performance assessment. At the present time there is no agreement on the content, timing, frequency, and type of examination. The purpose of this chapter is to present what constitutes a complete preparticipation evaluation.

Present Status of Preparticipation Evaluation

Feinstein and associates[2] surveyed the state high-school athletic associations of all 50 states and the District of Columbia. Table 1 shows the variations in state guidelines in several areas: frequency of examination, use of examination guidelines, use of medical history guidelines, recommendations for exclusion, use of parental consent forms for emergency treatment, and personnel authorized to do examinations. Through cooperation, national and state high-school associations and medical organizations can set standards and eliminate differences.

The Examination

Objectives   The preparticipation evaluation should have the following objectives[3-6]: (1) to determine the general health of the athlete; (2) to detect any conditions that might limit the athlete's participation; (3) to detect conditions that might predispose the athlete to injury (such as untreated injuries or illness, lack of conditioning, or congenital or developmental problems); (4) to assess the athlete's level of maturity; (5) to evaluate the athlete's fitness level; (6) to afford an opportunity for physician-athlete contact, so the physician can counsel the athlete about health and answer any health-related questions; and (7) to meet legal and insurance requirements.

Table 1. Variation in State Requirements for Preparticipation Examination

Guidelines for Participation	Required by States
Frequency of Exam	
Yearly	78% (35)
Every 3 years	7% (3)
Entry-level	2% (1)
No requirement	13% (6)
Official State Form	
Yes	80% (36)
No	20% (9)
Exam Guidelines	
Yes	62% (28)
No	38% (9)
Medical History	
Yes	56% (25)
No	44% (20)
Recommendations for Exclusion	
Yes	7% (3)
No	93% (42)
Parental Consent for Emergency Treatment	
Yes	44% (20)
No	56% (25)
Authorized to Give Exam	
Physician (MD)	34
MD/DO	4
MD/Certified Nurse Practitioner	1
MD/DO/Physician's Assistant	1
MD/DO/CNP/PA	1
Health Care Professional	1
Not Specified	3

Reproduced with permission from Feinstein RA, Soileau EJ, Daniel WJ: A national survey of preparticipation physical examination requirements. *Phys Sports Med* 1988;16:51-59.

Timing   The ideal time to conduct preparticipation physical examinations is six weeks before the season begins. This allows enough time to detect, correct, and/or rehabilitate any problems.[3,4]

Frequency   Although there are great variations among state requirements, yearly examinations are the most popular.[2] Young athletes are generally healthy. Four studies showed that only 3.2% to 13.5% of athletes needed rehabilitation and only 0.3% to 1.3% of athletes were disqualified.[5,7-9] Since 63% to 74% of problems can be identified through the medical history,[7,10] an entry-level history and thorough physical examination followed thereafter by an annual history and limited physical examination should be sufficient.

Type   The preparticipation physical examination can be done on an individual basis in the primary-care physician's office, or on a group basis through a station-type mass examination. Both offer distinct advantages.

Table 2. Station Examination

Activity	Person Responsible
Sign in	Athletic director or coach
Review history	Physician
Height/Weight	Coach
Visual acuity	Coach, nurse
Vital signs	Nurse
Medical examination	Physician
Orthopaedic examination	Physician
Review/reassessment	Physician
Body composition	Physiologist
Flexibility	Therapist or trainer
Strength	Therapist, coach, athletic trainer
Speed	Coach
Agility	Coach
Power	Coach
Balance	Coach
Endurance	Coach

If the evaluation takes place in the primary-care physician's office, there are the advantages of physician-patient familiarity and continuity of care. The physician has a complete history and medical records, and the privacy of an office setting provides the opportunity to discuss sensitive issues.

The components of a station-type mass examination appear in Table 2. With this approach, more specialized personnel (sports-oriented physicians, athletic trainers, physical therapists, dietitians, and exercise physiologists) can be included, and performance testing can be done. In addition, it offers time and cost efficiencies. The advantages of both can be obtained if the local primary-care physician participates and a private room for the evaluation is available in the station-type examination.

Medical History   The medical history is the keystone of any medical examination since it can help identify 63% to 74% of all problems.[7,10] Important subjects to explore in the history are hospitalizations and surgery, medication, allergies, tetanus status, the cardiovascular system and family history of cardiovascular problems, musculoskeletal system, neurologic system, dermatologic system, heat problems, other medical problems, and, for girls, menstrual history. A sample history form is shown in Appendix 1.

Risser and associates[10] showed that when medical history forms are completed separately by athletes and by their parents, only 39% of the forms matched. Therefore, it is very important to make the history forms available to the athletes before the examination so that their parents can help complete the form.

Physical Examination   During the physical examination, the areas of greatest concern and those identified as problems in the history can be emphasized and evaluated. A sample form is shown in Appendix 2. The examination should include height, weight, visual acuity, cardiovascular testing, blood pressure (130/75 in those under 10 years old and 140/85 in those 10 years old or older), pulses (radial, femoral), heart (rhythm, murmurs, size), musculoskeletal system, the abdominal system (organomegaly), skin (impetigo, acne, scabies, herpes, nevi), genitalia (single or undescended testicle, testicular mass), and maturity (Tanner staging).[11]

In the musculoskeletal section, a complete examination should be performed on any area identified as a problem by the history or the physical. A physical examination should be performed before the child enters middle school or high school. On a yearly basis, a cardiovascular examination (blood pressure, pulse, heart), skin examination, and maturity evaluation should be done, with a check on any potential problem area noted in the history.

Performance Testing

Performance testing can inform the athlete and the coach of the player's fitness. Fitness may help in injury prevention, although this has never been proven.

Performance tests can be done in a general fashion or in a more directed, sports-specific fashion, such as evaluating the flexibility and strength of a thrower's shoulders. Methods of performance evaluation[12-14] include body composition (skin folds, underwater weighing), flexibility (sit and reach, goniometric tests), strength (manual muscle testing, bench press/leg press, pull-ups, situps/pushups, isokinetics), endurance (12-minute run, 1.5-mile run), power (vertical jump, standing broad jump), speed (40-yard dash), sustained speed (440-yard run), agility (Illinois agility run), balance (stork stand), and dynamic balance (bass dynamic balance test, Springfield-Bram walking test).

The results of performance tests must be returned and explained to both coaches and athletes in a timely fashion.

Clearance

Based on the results of the physical examination, the physician can approve an athlete's participation in sports. This clearance can be divided into three categories:

1. Unrestricted participation in any type of sport, including contact-and-collision sports, limited-contact impact sports, and strenuous, moderately strenuous, and nonstrenuous noncontact sports.

2. Participation approved after coach, athletic trainer, and team physician have been notified about the child's problem.

3. Participation not approved until further evaluation is done by a physician.

Approval for participation should be based on specific guidelines. Recently, the American Academy of Pediatrics published recommendations for participation in competitive sports.[15] In addition the American

Table 3. Classification of Activities*

Contact		Noncontact		
Collision	Impact	Strenuous	Moderately Strenuous	Nonstrenuous
Boxing	Baseball	Aerobics	Badminton	Archery
Field hockey	Basketball	Crew	Curling	Golf
Football	Bicycling	Fencing	Table tennis	Riflery
Ice hockey	Diving	Discus		
Lacrosse	High jump	Javelin		
Martial arts	Pole vault	Shot put		
Rodeo	Gymnastics	Running		
Soccer	Riding horses	Swimming		
Wrestling	Ice skating	Tennis		
	Roller skating	Track		
	Skiing—	Weightlifting		
	cross-country			
	downhill			
	water			
	Softball			
	Squash, handball			
	Volleyball			

* Adapted with permission from American Academy of Pediatrics, Committee on Sports Medicine: Recommendations for participating in competitive sports. *Pediatrics* 1988;81:737-739.

Academy of Pediatrics' sports classification system [15] accurately classifies sports activities for participation approval (Table 3). These recommendations and classifications can guide the physician when helping an athlete choose an appropriate activity.

Summary

Since the preparticipation evaluation is an important preventive examination for the student athlete, a systematic approach is worthwhile. The most effective approach seems to be a complete entry-level evaluation with follow-up history and specific limited physical examination based on the history. The specific format for the preparticipation evaluation is an area of controversy and is best left to the individual situation and the preference of the examiner. More consistent guidelines for preparticipation evaluation from the responsible governing bodies for school sport are needed.

References

1. Crain TT (ed): *Comments in Sports Medicine*. Chicago, American Medical Association, 1973.
2. Feinstein RA, Soileau EJ, Daniel WJ: A national survey of preparticipation physical examination requirements. *Phys Sportsmed* 1988;16:51-59.
3. McKeag DB: Preseason physical exmination for the prevention of sports injuries. *Sports Med* 1985;2:413-431.

4. Lombardo JA: Pre-participation physical evaluation. *Primary Care* 1984; 11:3-21.

5. Linder CW, DuRant RH, Seklecki RM, et al: Preparticipation health screening of young athletes: Results of 1268 examinations. *Am J Sports Med* 1981;9:187-193.

6. Shaffer TE: The health examination for participation in sports. *Pediatr Ann* 1978;7:666-675.

7. Goldberg B, Saraniti A, Witman P, et al: Pre-participation sports assessment: An objective evaluation. *Pediatrics* 1980;66:736-745.

8. Thompson TR, Andrish JT, Bergfeld JA: A prospective study of preparticipation sports examinations for 2,670 young athletes: Method and results. *Cleve Clin Q* 1982;49:225-233.

9. Tennant FS Jr, Sorenson K, Day CM: Benefits of preparticipation sports examination. *J Fam Pract* 1981;13:287-288.

10. Risser WL, Hoffman HM, Bellah GG Jr: Frequency of preparticipation sports examinations in secondary school athletes: Are the University Interscholastic League guidelines appropriate? *Tex Med* 1985;81:35-39.

11. Smith N: *For the Practitioner: Orthopaedic Screening Examination for Participation in Sports.* Columbus, Ohio, Ross Laboratories, 1981.

12. Bosco JS, Gustafson WF: *Measurement and Evaluation in Physical Education, Fitness and Sports.* Englewood Cliffs, Prentice-Hall, 1983.

13. Johnson BL, Nelson JK: *Practical Measurement for Evaluation in Physical Education.* Edina, Minnesota, Burgess Publishing, 1974.

14. Cooper KH: A means of assessing maximal oxygen uptake: Correlation between field and treadmill testing. *JAMA* 1968;203:201-204.

15. American Academy of Pediatrics, Committee on Sports Medicine: Recommendations for participation in competitive sports. *Pediatrics* 1988;81:737-739.

Appendix I

History Form

Name _____   Date of Birth _____

Address _____   Class _____

Parents _____   Phone # _____

Physician _____

Sports _____   _____

Fill in details of "YES" answers in space below:

		Yes	No
1.	Have you ever been hospitalized?	___	___
	Have you ever had surgery?	___	___
2.	Are you presently taking medication?	___	___
3.	Do you have any allergies (medicines, bees)?	___	___
4.	Have you ever passed out during exercise?	___	___
	Have you ever been dizzy during exercise?	___	___
	Have you ever had chest pain?	___	___
	Do you tire more quickly than your friends during exercise?	___	___
	Have you ever had high blood pressure?	___	___
	Have you ever been told you have a heart murmur?	___	___
	Have you ever had racing of your heart or skipped beats?	___	___
	Has anyone in your family died of heart problems or died suddenly before age 40?	___	___
5.	Do you have any skin problems? (itching, moles, breaking out)	___	___
6.	Have you ever had a head injury?	___	___
	Have you ever been knocked out?	___	___
	Have you ever had a seizure?	___	___
	Have you ever had a stinger or burner?	___	___
7.	Have you ever injured (sprained, dislocated, fractured, etc.):		

_____ Hand   _____ Shoulder   _____ Thigh

_____ Wrist   _____ Neck   _____ Knee

_____ Forearm   _____ Chest   _____ Shin/Calf

_____ Elbow   _____ Back   _____ Ankle

_____ Arm   _____ Hip   _____ Foot

8.   Have you ever had heat cramps?   _____   _____

Have you ever been dizzy or passed out in the heat?   _____   _____

9.   Have you ever had:

_____ Mononucleosis   _____ Diabetes

_____ Hepatitis   _____ Headaches (frequent)

_____ Asthma   _____ Eye injuries

_____ Tuberculosis   _____ Stomach ulcer

10.   Do you use special pads or braces?   _____   _____

11.   When was your last tetanus shot? _____

(Girls only)

12.   When was your first menstrual period? _____

When was your last menstrual period? _____

Explain YES answers here:

_____

_____

_____

_____

_____

_____

Parent's signature: _____

Appendix 2

Physical Examination

Height _____   Weight _____   BP _____   Pulse _____

Visual acuity   _____

CV Pulses   _____

    Heart   _____

Abdominal   _____

Skin   _____

Genitalia   _____

Tanner   _____

Musculoskeletal   _____

    Neck   _____

    Shoulder   _____

    Elbow   _____

    Wrist   _____

    Hand   _____

    Back   _____

    Knee   _____

    Ankle   _____

    Foot   _____

Assessment _____

_____

_____

_____

_____

Recommendation _____

_____

_____

_____

_____

Chaper 10

Chronic Illness

Michael Nelson, MD

Introduction

Children with chronic diseases often benefit from increased levels of activity. Sports precautions need to be evaluated on a case-by-case basis, to be sure the proposed activity is appropriate and that precautions are taken prior to participation, e.g., correct medications, diet, etc. Patients with chronic diseases of childhood should be encouraged to participate in sport activity at a level commensurate with their condition. Chronic dependency should not be fostered between the parent and family. In 1986 and 1987, the American Academy of Pediatrics Sports Medicine Committee[1] revised the American Medical Association's 12-year-old guidelines[2] on participation in sports by athletes with chronic illnesses. This revision was necessary for several reasons. In some cases, previous guidelines were thought to be overly restrictive, especially as the rights of the individual to engage in risk-taking activity have broadened in society. The quality of medical care and understanding of sports-medicine issues have also improved. Rule changes and equipment modifications may lessen the risks undertaken by an individual sports participant with chronic disease.[3]

New diseases have been identified since 1976 and previously unknown ramifications of some chronic illnesses have been recognized. Individual practitioners also needed more latitude in making decisions with their patients about participation in sports.

This chapter focuses on the revised guidelines for participation in sports by individuals with chronic disease. It also examines the new guidelines for conditions that were not previously identified as presenting potential problems in sports.

Hypertension

In the 1976 guidelines, hypertension on an "organic basis" precluded participation in any sport. Since then, studies have shown that aerobic exercise has a beneficial effect on the clinical course of hypertension.[4] Strength training, weightlifting, or any sport using the Valsalva's maneuver may result in dramatic elevation of blood pressure (>300 mm Hg systolic) in individuals with moderate or severe hypertension.[4] The clinical significance of these elevations is unknown. The usefulness of exercise stress testing for athletes with moderate or severe hypertension has not been determined. There is no convincing evidence that those with mild hypertension are at risk in any sport; however, a stress test should be performed on athletes with mildly-increased blood pressure who become symptomatic (that is, experience dizziness, chest pain, or syncope) during exercise. There is a sound basis for the belief that aerobic exercise has a therapeutic effect on weight control, blood lipid patterns, and blood pressure.[5-7] Aerobic exercise prescriptions should be a part of the therapy for any hypertensive patient.

Convulsive Disorders

With the availability of newer therapies for treating convulsive disorders and a better understanding of the natural history of these diseases, it is now appropriate to allow individuals with controlled seizures to participate in any sport; however, some controversy still exists. Hulse and Strong[8] recommend that children with psychomotor seizures be excluded from strenuous noncontact and contact sports.

Seizures are unlikely to occur during sports participation, but individuals who have poorly-controlled epilepsy should probably avoid contact and limited-contact sports, as well as swimming, weightlifting, shooting, and archery. Exercise has not been shown to improve seizure control.

Hernia

Previously, the presence of a hernia precluded athletic participation in virtually all sports. There is no evidence that participation in a sport leads to an increase in the rate of incarceration. After appropriate counseling of the athlete, a physician may choose to delay closure of a hernia until the end of the competitive season.

Asthma

The incidence of pulmonary tuberculosis has declined over the years and is no longer included in the guidelines. Asthma, however, is being diagnosed more frequently. Asthmatics can now participate in all sports because of medical therapy not available 12 years ago. Athletes with severe respiratory insufficiency (such as cystic fibrosis) should have an exercise stress test to determine their oxygen-desaturation threshold before they participate in anything other than nonstrenuous sports.[4]

Exercise-induced asthma occurs in about 12% of the general population and in the majority of asthmatics. Inhaling beta-agonists or cromolyn sodium before exercise is an effective preventive treatment.[2] Exercising in warm, humid environments (as in an indoor pool), nasal breathing, and short repetitive exercise periods are ways to lessen the severity of exercise-induced asthma.[4]

Using exercise in asthma therapy is beneficial in a number of ways. Although there is no significant evidence that exercise improves pulmonary function, it improves fitness levels, endurance, VO_2 max, and school attendance, and lessens the severity of emotional lability and of asthma not related to exercise.[8]

Diabetes Mellitus Type I

Exercise has the same beneficial effects for diabetics that it has for everyone. Exercise improves both plasma-lipid profiles and respiratory- and cardiac-fitness parameters.[9] Attempts to show that exercise improves diabetic control, as measured by glycosylated-hemoglobin levels, have met with mixed results. Most researchers have not found any reductions in glycosylated hemoglobin in response to exercise programs, but there has been at least one controversial study demonstrating such a relationship. Even if diabetic control is not improved, the other benefits of exercise support the removal of diabetes as a contraindication for sports participation.

The diabetic athlete must be managed carefully. An injection site in the most actively utilized body parts will increase the absorption of insulin (that is, insulin injected into the thigh of a runner is more rapidly absorbed). Caloric intake must increase in proportion to the intensity of the activity to be performed. Timing caloric intake to occur just before exercise can help prevent hypoglycemia. The concept of "exercise exchanges" may be useful in balancing energy intake and output and in preventing wide variations in glucose homeostasis.[4]

Down Syndrome

The recognition of atlantoaxial instability in individuals with Down syndrome has prompted the development of guidelines for sports participation by these youngsters. The American Academy of Pediatrics recommends that children with Down syndrome have a roentgenogram of the neck in neutral, flexion, and extension positions before participating in sports. If the distance between the odontoid process of the axis and the anterior arch of the atlas exceeds 4.5 mm or if the odontoid is abnormal, participation in sports that involve trauma to the head and neck should be restricted. If there is subluxation or dislocation and neurologic signs, all strenuous activities should be restricted and surgical stabilization should be considered. If there is no evidence of instability, the individual may participate in all sports and no follow-up is required.[10]

A recent review of the data used to develop these guidelines has questioned the validity of the recommendations,[11] particularly regarding the need for and frequency of radiologic evaluation in the asymptomatic individual. Neurologic symptoms and signs are almost always present for extended periods before any injury is documented. It may be that the current guidelines are overly restrictive. Fifteen to thirty percent of persons with Down syndrome have the radiographic criteria of instability, not all of whom have or ever develop neurologic deficits. When both are present, surgical stabilization is indicated.

Both the radiographic and neurologic findings can change with time, so that these patients need sequential follow-up. No long-term controlled studies are available to document the natural history of this condition. It may be that when the patient is asymptomatic, the importance of radiographic findings has been overemphasized. Therefore, the current recommendation that asymptomatic patients with radiographic findings be prohibited from participating in at-risk sports may be overly restrictive. Long-term controlled studies are needed to document present belief.

What then should the practitioner recommend? All children with Down syndrome should be periodically evaluated for cervical instability. Around the age of five, the child should have a neurologic examination and a set of flexion/extension lateral radiographs. These examinations should be repeated every two to three years. Those whose neurologic and radiographic examinations are normal should not have their activity restricted. On radiograph, if the atlanto-dens interval is greater than 6 mm, the child should be prohibited from participating in any sport that stresses the cervical spine. Patients with neurologic deficit require consideration for stabilization.

Sickle Cell Trait

Military recruits with sickle cell trait have a higher rate of sudden death than those without the trait.[12] The deaths occur almost exclusively during basic training. There is no evidence of sudden death among athletes with the sickle cell trait. At present, there is no evidence to suggest that athletes with the sickle-cell trait should be excluded from sports participation. These and all other athletes should pay proper attention to good hydration and allow adequate time for acclimatization to heat and altitude changes.

Acquired Immune Deficiency Syndrome

Since the development of the guidelines, there has been some controversy regarding sports participation by athletes with acquired immune deficiency syndrome (AIDS).

Potential exposure of athletes to the AIDS virus as well as the participation of athletes with AIDS in sports are emotionally charged and controversial issues. There is no evidence that the AIDS virus can be spread by athletic competition. Body secretions should be handled according to the guidelines developed by the Centers for Disease Control.[13] The epidemiology of this disease needs to be better understood before sound and rational guidelines can be developed for sports participation by the athlete with AIDS. At this time, the only appropriate recommendations are those regarding the handling of body secretions.

References

1. American Academy of Pediatrics, Committee on Sports Medicine: Participation in competitive sports. *Pediatrics* 1988;81:737-739.
2. American Medical Association: *Medical Evaluation of the Athlete: A Guide*, rev ed. Chicago, American Medical Association, 1976.
3. American Academy of Pediatrics, Committee on Sports Medicine: *Sports Medicine: Health Care for Young Athletes.* Elk Grove Village, Illinois, American Academy of Pediatrics, 1985.
4. Bar-Or O: *Pediatric Sports Medicine for the Practitioner.* New York, Springer-Verlag, 1983.
5. Hagberg JM, Eshani AA, Goldring D, et al: Effect of weight training on blood pressure and hemodynamics in hypertensive adolescents. *J of Pediatrics* 1984; 104:147-151.
6. Podolsky ML: Don't rule out sports for hypertensive children. *The Physician and Sports Medicine.* 1989; 17:164-170.
7. Frohlich ED, Lowenthall DT, Miller HS, et al: Systemic Arterial Hypertension. *Jour Am College of Cardiology* 1985;6:1218-1221.
8. Hulse E, Strong WB: Preparticipation evaluation in athletes. *Pediatr Rev* 1987; 9:1-10.
9. Blackett PR: Child and adolescent athletes with diabetes. *Phys Sports Med* 1988;16:133-149.
10. American Academy of Pediatrics, Committee on Sports Medicine: Atlantoaxial instability in Down syndrome. *Pediatrics* 1984;74:152-154.
11. Davidson RG: Atlantoaxial instability in individuals with Down syndrome: A fresh look at the evidence. *Pediatrics* 1988;81:857-865.
12. Kark JA, Posey PM, et al: Sickle cell trait as a risk factor for sudden death in physical training. *New Engl J Med* 1987;317:781-787.
13. *Guidelines for Health Care Workers for Prevention of AIDS.* Atlanta, Centers for Disease Control, 1988.

Chapter 11

The Young Female Athlete

Letha Y. Hunter-Griffin, MD, PhD

The Female Athlete

Title IX has resulted in an explosion of participation in women's sport. Many girls and young women come to the athletic arena with limited presport conditioning, which commonly results in rapid acquisition of a myriad of overuse problems. Improved coaching awareness regarding conditioning, equipment, and rules will enhance female sport participation while reducing risk of injury.

Injuries in women's sports are sport-specific and not sex-specific. Injuries continue to be manifested as sequelae of macrotrauma, e.g., fractures, sprains, strains, and microtrauma. This latter genre is commonly secondary to overuse of the underused. Progressive conditioning programs and appropriate conditioning drills and techniques will help eliminate many of the conditions in this stress-related category.

The Changing Abilities of the Female Athlete During Development

The young female athlete goes through the three stages of development—childhood, adolescence, and young adulthood. Adolescence is also called the pubertal period, childhood is the prepubertal period, and young adulthood is the postpubertal period. Athletic abilities differ in each stage.

Boys and girls are most equal in their athletic abilities during childhood. This is the time for equal and same competition. In most grade schools, gym classes include soccer, basketball, softball, and baseball, with boys and girls participating together up until the sixth grade. Then, at about age 12, pubertal development alters this balance. Of course, puberty is a continuum, and not everyone reaches the same stage at the same time. Boys go through puberty at about 13 to 15 years of age, while girls experience it at 11 to 13 years of age.

During the pubertal years, schools and leagues should consider basing programs on weight rather than age. If two girls are both 13 years old, but one has gone through puberty and the other is just starting, their sizes will be very different. This size difference can be of even greater significance in prepubertal and postpubertal boys.

After puberty, there are differences between males and females that were not present in childhood. Males increase in height, weight, and muscle mass. Although females also increase in height and weight, they do so to a lesser degree than males. Moreover, there is no parallel increase in muscle mass. Most postpubertal males are taller, heavier, and stronger than females of the same age.

Although the postpubescent female has less muscle mass than her male counterpart, she generally has a greater amount of body fat per total body weight.[1] In equally-conditioned men and women, muscle is 23% of a woman's body weight, whereas it is 40% of a man's body weight. Women have 15% body fat, compared with 5% in men.[2] Thus, women are at a slight physiologic disadvantage in sports, with less muscle mass to carry more weight.

Physiologic parameters also differ. Postpubertal females have smaller hearts, smaller rib cages, smaller vital capacities, and greater respiratory rates than equally-conditioned postpubertal males.[3] So, although childhood abilities are similar, puberty brings marked differences in athletic potential between the sexes. At this stage, the aim of sport participation for boys and girls should be equal opportunity but not necessarily coeducational participation.[4]

The postpubertal female athlete may find it more difficult to continue to compete with her male counterpart. In addition, she may find it difficult to excel in some sports in which she previously participated. That is, she may "grow out" of her sport.

For example, if a young, thin, elite gymnast finds that her body physique is significantly altered during pubertal development, she may find it difficult to continue at her previous level of proficiency. Similarly, a star ballerina who develops a large bust during puberty may find she no longer has the lean, sleek look that is expected of her.

These girls may feel frustrated if they continue to pursue a sport in which they are no longer comfortable or confident, but they may not be able to express this frustration to their parents. The girls know how much time and effort their parents have devoted to their sport development. They know their parents look forward to their continued participation. Young girls in this situation may try to "escape" participating by complaining of numerous minor injuries. They may feel frustrated or depressed. Physicians evaluating these athletes for their many minor complaints should be sensitive to the larger problem. The physician may need to be an intermediary between teenager and parent, by explaining to the parent that these young women may no longer fit their sport, cannot perform at their previous level of achievement, and would rather withdraw from the sport than continue to be frustrated by diminished performance.

Psychological, as well as physical, development during puberty may cause a female athlete to grow out of her sport. Although ideas are changing, boys have traditionally proven their masculinity through sport participation, while girls, especially those involved in contact sports, have had to prove their femininity.[5] For teenagers, these psychological demands come at a crucial time, just as they are trying to find themselves and their place in the world. In addition to this perception factor, there are also time limitations. Teenage girls typically begin to pay more attention to their appearance and to experiment with hairstyles, make-up, and clothes. They may no longer want to spend every night in the gym.

Advantages of Continued Sport Participation

For young women, continued participation in sports as they grow offers many advantages. It is more acceptable today for women to be tall, tough, and competitive. Fathers are teaching sport skills to their daughters as well as to their sons, thus forming closer father-daughter relationships. Many people also believe that increased "team" participation by young women will help them succeed in business in the future.

The Preparticipation Physical Examination

The preseason screening examination should be adapted to address special areas of concern to female athletes. Additional points should be considered in each aspect of the examination.

Family History   An athlete's medical history includes a family history. When screening female athletes, a physician should ask about scoliosis since there is a familial tendency to this spinal deformity. Scoliosis is more common in women, who also tend to have greater curve progression.[6] If a girl has a family history of scoliosis, she should be monitored very carefully during her rapid growth years (ages 11 to 13 years).

A family history of cardiovascular disease is also important to note, especially in the college and elite athlete. Although coronary artery disease is more common in men, premenopausal women can be affected.[1,7] Elite athletes, performing at maximum levels, may need to have stress electrocardiograms as early as the late teens, if there is a strong family history of arteriosclerotic heart disease.

Mitral valve prolapse, another condition that runs in families, is also more common among women. It can be diagnosed when a mid-systolic click, associated with a late systolic murmur, is heard and confirmed by an echocardiogram. Typically, this condition alone does not preclude sports participation. However, further investigation is warranted if it is associated with syncope, disabling chest pain, complex ventricular arrhythmias, significant mitral regurgitation, prolonged QT interval, Marfan's syndrome, or a family history of sudden death.[8]

Medical History   It is important to include questions on the urogenital system when reviewing the medical history of a female athlete. If a woman has a history of urinary tract infections, the physician should discuss the need for frequent fluid intake, especially water. Some athletes tend to diminish their fluid intake when traveling, and should be cautioned not to do so.

The physician should document the date of first menses, the date of the last period, the average length of the period, the presence of dysmenorrhea, and any pregnancy history. Athletes may have delayed menarche. Nonathletes experience menarche at an average age of 12.5 years, while for athletes the average age is 13.5 to 15.5 years.[9]

The athlete who has not had a period by 16 years of age is considered to have primary amenorrhea. She should be referred to her physician for further evaluation to determine the reason for the delayed menstrual periods.[10]

The normal menstrual cycle is 28 days, with a range of 25 to 35 days.[9] Many athletes (as many as 46% of runners) have oligomenorrhea, or infrequent periods (cycles longer than 35 days, but shorter than 90 days).[11] Secondary amenorrhea, or cessation of menses for longer than three months, is reported by 5% to 15% of athletes.[1] Secondary amenorrhea is more common in sports such as running and activities such as ballet, and less common in sports such as swimming and cycling.[12]

Physical stress, emotional stress, and weight loss appear to be major factors contributing to the development of secondary amenorrhea. Athletes who have not had a menstrual period in a year should not assume that their amenorrhea is caused by their athletic participation. They should be evaluated to exclude other abnormalities.[1]

Some gynecologists advocate estrogen replacement in low-estrogen secondary amenorrhea. They believe that prolonged low-estrogen states may result in early osteoporosis.

Cann and others noted a decrease in the cancellous bone of the vertebral bodies in female athletes amenorrheic for a year or longer. The amount of cortical bone did not change, and the significance of the cancellous bone loss is not clear.[13] Estrogen replacement does have consequences and side effects. Moreover, many female athletes have a psychological aversion to replacement therapy, even if it is recommended.

Contraceptive methods can be discussed as part of the menstrual history. Girls need to be reminded that secondary amenorrhea is no guarantee against pregnancy. The amenorrheic athlete may start ovulating normally at any time. Most athletes do not like to take birth control pills, but those who do take them should not use them to regulate their periods around major competitions.

Dysmenorrhea, or painful period, is less common in athletes than in nonathletes. If it does occur, dysmenorrhea can be disabling to the athlete during competition. Menstrual cramps are caused by endometrial release of prostaglandins, which then act on the myometrium and cause contractions.

Prostaglandin inhibitors such as naproxen sodium, ibuprofen, and naproxen may be used to treat dysmenorrhea. Persistent, disabling dysmenorrhea deserves further gynecologic evaluation to rule out endometriosis, pelvic infection, and other diseases.

Frequent vaginal infections should also be noted. If antibiotics must be used in athletes susceptible to *Candida* vaginitis, the physician may recommend preventive douches or medicated suppositories to avoid future infections.

Physical Examination

Cardiovascular System   The physician should place particular emphasis on listening to the midsystolic click and late systolic murmur of mitral valve prolapse, since mitral valve prolapse occurs with greater frequency in women. It is by no means limited to women, however. If the preparticipation screen uncovers a midsystolic click previously unknown to the athlete, the orthopaedist may wish to refer the athlete to her physician for further evaluation. Prophylactic antibiotics should be given to athletes with mitral valve prolapse in the event of severe abrasions, dental work, or gastrointestinal instrumentation.[14]

Breast Examination   Including a breast examination as part of a preparticipation physical depends on the age of the athlete. For college and older athletes, a breast examination should be done if this will be the athlete's only physical. However, if the preparticipation physical examination is a sport-specific examination to augment a routine physical done by a private physician, there is no need to do a breast examination. If the athlete is very large-breasted, the physician can counsel her on the use of sports bras.

Pelvic Examination   Most physicians do not do pelvic examinations as part of preparticipation physicals. The exception is the family physician doing the preparticipation physical as part of a complete physical examination. If the medical history of an athlete reveals something unusual or abnormal about her menstrual history, the physician can refer the athlete to her physician for additional gynecologic evaluation.

Musculoskeletal Examination

Joint Laxity   Women have been reported to have greater joint laxity than men.[15] In preseason physicals, it is important to document the degree of laxity of major joints, including shoulders, knees (anteroposterior, medial-lateral, patellar laxity), and ankles. Then, if an injury occurs, the preinjury laxity is available for comparison. Furthermore, if the joint laxity exceeds age-related norms, preseason conditioning exercises can be developed to strengthen the muscles.

Spine   A physician should assess the cervical, thoracic, and lumbar spine. The physician should note the presence of excessive lumbar lordosis, scoliosis, or thoracic kyphosis. Certain sports, such as women's gymnastics, women's diving, roller skating, ice skating, and ballet, emphasize lumbar hyperextension. Girls participating in these sports should strengthen abdominal and paravertebral muscles to minimize the occurrence of lumbar pain and the potential for stress fractures of the pars interarticularis.

Knees   During the knee examination, the physician should note patellar laxity, as well as patellar tracking patterns during active and passive extension of the knee.

While the athlete is standing, the examiner should look at the configuration of the lower extremities as a whole. If femoral anteversion, foot pronation, and a laterally tracking patella are observed, the physician should recommend that the athlete's conditioning program include exercises to strengthen the quadriceps muscle and the vastus medialis fibers.

A supplemental biking program may be excellent for the female athlete with patellar pain or abnormal patellar tracking. Biking can increase quadriceps strength at low patellofemoral forces. The seat of the bicycle saddle should be maximally elevated and the tension low during the exercise. Women with subluxating or laterally tracking patellas, as well as those with parapatellar or retropatellar tenderness or evidence of patellar crepitation should avoid stair-climbing drills.

If the patella subluxates easily with gentle pressure on the medial side, a patella-stabilizing brace made with a lateral restraining pad may be helpful. This condition is unusual in junior college, college, or elite athletes, since it typically disables an athlete early in her career.

Foot   In examining the foot of the athlete, the physician should note soft or hard corns, or thickening of the bursa over the first metatarsal head medially, the fifth metatarsal head laterally, or over the superior prominence of the calcaneus posteriorly. Such findings usually indicate that the athlete is wearing an improperly-fitted shoe.

Many women have slender heels, but a proportionately wider forefoot. Shoes fitted to the hindfoot may be too narrow for the forefoot. Conversely, shoes wide enough for the forefoot may be too wide for the heel, causing the foot to slide forward in the shoe and impingement of the forefoot.

Foot pain caused by shoewear can be disabling to an athlete. Symptoms from bursitis, corns, and blisters are slow to resolve once they occur, so the emphasis must be on prevention.

Bunions are found more frequently in girls than in boys.[16] These are usually asymptomatic. However, if they are symptomatic, modifying the shoe should be tried initially rather than surgery. Surgical correction of bunions can alter foot mechanics and lead to other problems. Most bunionectomies shorten the first metatarsal, thus shifting the weight-bearing axis to the center of the foot. Stress fractures or metatarsalgia of the middle metatarsals can result.

Laboratory Tests   The preparticipation physical examination of the athlete in high school or junior high school rarely includes laboratory testing of blood or urine; the low yields of such testing do not make it cost-effective.[17] If the preparticipation physical is done by the athlete's physician as part of an annual examination, a blood count and urinalysis may be obtained.

Where financially feasible, iron levels should be obtained in addition to a hematocrit for the college-age female athlete. Tissue iron may be depleted before an athlete's hematocrit falls. Iron is important for both oxygen transport and oxidative enzyme function. Depleted iron stores may adversely affect performance by decreasing strength and endurance, resulting in easy fatigability. Altered visual perception has also been blamed on depleted tissue iron. Measuring serum ferritin levels is a reasonable way to assess tissue iron.[1]

Iron deficiencies have been reported in the basic diet of 50% of women. Physicians should counsel women to include iron-rich foods in their diets. These foods include meats (liver, oysters, turkey, pork, beef), dried fruits (apricots, dates, prunes, raisins), and beans (baked, lima, kidney, refried).[18]

Fitness Evaluation   Assessing physical fitness for both male and female athletes includes evaluating muscle strength, muscle power, speed, agility, flexibility, and cardiovascular endurance.[19]

In evaluating performance in the postpubertal athlete, the physician cannot use the same parameters to assess men and women's performances. After puberty anatomic and physiologic differences between the sexes influence results.[20]

Conditioning Techniques and Their Effect on Injury Rates

Many observers predicted an increase in the number and types of injuries as women became more aggressive and competitive in sports. In fact, early injury studies reported that female athletes sustained more injuries than male athletes.[21,22] As women became more serious about sports participation, however, they improved their training and conditioning techniques, and their injury rates have decreased.[23]

Injuries are more sport-specific than sex-specific. That is, injury types and rates are similar for men and women in the same sport, but differ for athletes participating in different sports.[24]

Conditioning programs help the athlete achieve strength, endurance, and flexibility and, hence, decrease the chance of injury. At one time, people feared that girls would become "muscle-bound" if they participated in weight-training programs as part of their conditioning programs. Results now show that weight training is beneficial to girls. It increases their strength and does not result in large increases in muscle bulk, unless the girl is genetically predisposed. Weight-training programs can increase a girl's strength by as much as to 40% without increasing muscle bulk.

Nutritional Concerns

After puberty, the basal metabolic rate is lower in women than in men.[25] Hence, women need fewer calories to sustain the same level of activity as their male counterparts. Nonetheless, all required dietary components must be included within these total calories.

Women athletes have a higher incidence of eating disorders (principally anorexia nervosa and bulimia) than men. Perhaps this is a result of the image changes puberty brings. The athlete may find her "new" body undesirable in sports such as track, ice skating, and ballet in which the lean look is appreciated, and respond with a change in eating habits.

Anorexia nervosa is a severe and prolonged inability or refusal to eat, sometimes accompanied by spontaneous or induced vomiting. Anorexia is more than simply starving oneself to "make weight." It is a psychological disorder in which the individual perceives herself as much heavier than is actually the case. Bulimia is the marked fear of becoming obese, with uncontrolled binges followed by purging, vomiting, laxatives, or excessive exercise.

Eating disorders have been estimated to occur in 13% to 17% of female athletes. Eating disorders occur primarily in the middle and upper classes and are nine times more common in females than males. The typical sufferer is 15 to 26 years of age.[26]

Girls with eating disorders may be more susceptible to injury and more likely to seek treatment from their orthopaedist. In fact, the orthopaedist may be the only physician this girl sees. It is important that the doctor recognize the scope of the illness and encourage the athlete and her parents to seek help. The parents may not even realize their child has an eating disorder, or, if they do, they may not know how to deal with it.

At the other extreme, some girls use anabolic steroids combined with protein diets and rigorous weight-training regimens to increase muscle bulk. These athletes should realize that anabolic steroids have serious side effects. Some side effects (acne or excess facial hair) are reversible when the athlete stops taking the drug. Other side effects, including menstrual irregularity, male-pattern baldness, deepening of the voice, enlarged clitoris, fluid retention, and increased blood pressure, cannot be reversed. The use of anabolic steroids should be condemned.

Conclusion

In summary then, the athletic abilities of young boys and girls may be equal. As they approach adolescence, however, boys and girls experience physical changes of puberty that affect their athletic abilities. Children, especially girls, may grow out of the sports for which they have been groomed. Psychological problems may be manifested as physical ailments. It then becomes the physician's responsibility to see beyond the superficial injury to the larger problem, and to help the athlete and her family seek solutions.

Conditioning is as important in girls as in boys, because proper conditioning decreases injury rates. Nutritional problems in teenage girls are more prevalent than in teenage boys, and need to be identified and addressed.

References

1. Wells C: *Women, Sport and Performance.* Human Kinetics, Champaign, 1985;7.
2. Puhl J, Brown C, Voy R: *Sport Science Perspectives for Women.* Human Kinetics, Champaign, 1988;13-21.

3. Klafs C, Lyon M: *The Female Athlete*. CV Mosby, St. Louis, 1978;15-29.

4. Albohm M: Equal but separate—ensuring safety in athletics. *J of the NATA* 1978;13:131-132.

5. Hunter L: Aspects of injuries to the lower extremity unique to the female athlete. In Nicholas J, Hershman E. *The Lower Extremity and Spine in Sports Medicine.* CV Mosby, St. Louis, 1986;96-97.

6. Loveall W, Winter R: *Pediatric Orthopaedics,* 2nd ed., vol. 2, Lippincott, Philadelphia, 1986;580.

7. Leon A: Cadiovascular considerations. In Haycock C (ed): *Sports Medicine for the Athletic Female.* Medical Economics, Oradell, 1980;117-125.

8. Jeresaty R: Mitral valve prolapse: definition and implications in athletes. *J of the Am Coll Cardiol* 1986;7(1):231-236.

9. Shangold M, Mirkin G: *The Complete Sports Medicine Book for Women.* Fireside Books, New York, 1985;138.

10. Shangold M: Gynecological and endocrinological factors. In Haycock C (ed): *Sports Medicine for the Athletic Female.* Medical Economics, Oradell, 1980;316-329.

11. Frisch R, Wyshak G, Vincent C: Delayed menarche and amenorrhea in ballet dancers. *N Eng J Med* 1980;303:17-19.

12. Sanborn C, Martin B, Wagner W: Is athletic amenorrhea specific to runners? *Am J Obstet Gynecol* 1982;143:859-861.

13. Cann C, Martin M, Genant H, et al: Decreased spinal mineral content in amenorrheic women. *JAMA* 1984;251(5):626-629.

14. Perloff J, Child J, Edwards J: New guidelines for the clinical diagnosis of mitral valvle prolapse. *Amer J Cardiol* 1986;57:1124-1129.

15. Powers J: *Title IX Knee.* American Academy of Orthopaedic Surgeons Hilton Head Symposium, April, 1977.

16. Hunter L: Women's athletics: the orthopaedic surgeon's viewpoint. *Clin in Sports Med* 1984;3(4):809-827.

17. Runyan D: The preparticipation examination of the young athlete: defining the essentials. *Clin Pediatr* 1983;22(10):674-679.

18. Smith N: *Food for Sport.* Bull Publishing, Palo Alto, 1976;105-113.

19. Blum R: Preparticipation evaluation of the adolescent athlete. *Postgrad Med* 1985;78(2):52-69.

20. Gaillard B, Haskell W, Smith N, Ogilvie B: *Handbook for the Young Athlete.* Bull Publishing, Palo Alto, 1978;36-37.

21. Eisenberg I, Allen W: Injuries in a women's varsity athletics program. *Phys and Sportsmed* 1979;(7):5-11.

22. Kosek S: *Nature and incidence of women in sports.* National Sports Safety Congress, Cincinnati, OH, Feb, 1973;50-53.

23. Clarke K, Buckley W: Women's injuries in collegiate sports. *Amer J of Sports Med* 1979;7:138-144.

24. Whiteside P: Men's and women's injuries in comparable sports. *Phys and Sportsmed* 1980;8:130-140.

25. Hunter L, Andrews J, Clancy W, et al: Common orthopaedic problems of female athletes, in Frankel VH (ed): American Academy of Orthopaedic Surgeons *Instructional Course Lectures, XXXI.* St. Louis, CV Mosby, 1982, pp 126-151.

26. Eating disorders in young athletes: a round table. *Phys and Sportsmed,* 1985;13(11):89-106.

Additional Readings

Birrell S: Discourses on the gender/sport relationship: from women in sport to gender relations. In Pandolf K ed. *Exercise and Sport Sciences Reviews,* vol. 16, MacMillan, New York, 1988;459-502.

Clark N, Nelson M, Evans W: Nutrition education for elite female runners. *Phys and Sportsmed* 1988;16(2):124-136.

Drinkwater B: ed. *Female Endurance Athletes* Human Kinetics, Champaign, 1986.

Ellison A: ed. *Athletic Training and Sports Medicine*. American Academy of Orthopaedic Surgeons, Park Ridge, 1984;465-472.

Rosen L, McKeag D, Hough D, Curley V: Pathogenic wight-control behaviour in female atheltes. *Phys and Sportsmed* 1986;14(1):79-86.

Shangold M, Mirkin G: Women and Exercise. *Physiol and Sports Med* Davis FA, Philadelphia, 1988.

Sports Psychology and Organization

Chapter 12

The Role of the Pediatric Sports Medicine Specialist in Youth Sports

Bruce C. Ogilvie, PhD

Introduction

Although physicians understand the importance of being fit, they have been unable to change the beliefs and attitudes of the general public about personal fitness. Surveys over the past two decades confirm that 50% of adults have a sedentary lifestyle. Yet children are by nature active creatures who engage in spontaneous games and play. They need only an environment conducive to such behavior and positive reinforcement from adults. How, then, is this most natural of all behavior gradually extinguished between the ages of 4 and 16 years? What are the major factors contributing to the high attrition rate in youth sports?

One reason is the failure of adults to let children determine how to best meet their fitness needs. Rarely are fitness activities truly child-centered but tend to center around organized sports. Solving this problem requires an examination of the social and psychological needs of children in recreation and sport.

Sports physicians must take a more active role in educating adults involved in youth sports. Few coaches have any formal training for such a responsible role. Actual film footage in the documentary "Youth Sports, Who's Really Competing?" shows that coaches model themselves after television images and that their coaching behaviors are more appropriate for adults than for children. Physicians can make a significant contribution to the welfare of children in sports if they take greater responsibility for developing and training coaches.

Educating parents about their appropriate role in their child's recreational or competitive activities is often neglected. Parental attitudes and behavior are tied to a child's continued participation and to the child's ability to grow and benefit from sports. Parental attitude is one of the most powerful positive influences in developing a fitness or sports ethic.

Recreation and sport have also failed to provide for the needs of millions of physically disadvantaged children. In the last decade, research on elite disabled athletes has created a knowledge base and provided some generalizations about the social, psychological, and physical needs of these children. These data must be used to educate and interest communities so that equal opportunities are available for these underserved children.

The Case for the Importance of Fitness

The fitness wave that swept the United States during the past decade has not changed the attitudes and behavior of children. A 1984 study by the American Athletic Union reported that only 36% of schoolchildren met the criteria of average fitness.[1] The fact that 40% of 6- to 15-year-old boys cannot touch their toes indicates serious disregard for the importance of flexibility. The U.S. Public Health Service reported that one-third of American youths are not physically active enough to experience an aerobic benefit.

Many degenerative diseases have their roots in negative habits and behaviors formed during early childhood. Studies done in Michigan and Nebraska found that 40% of the elementary-school children tested showed one of the primary risk factors for future heart disease: increased blood cholesterol level, high blood pressure, obesity, and poor cardiac fitness.[2]

In cross-cultural comparisons of youth fitness based on international standards, the typical American child is a poor performer. Various studies rank American children in the lower 20% of developed nations. Although these findings have been consistent for the past 20 years, they have apparently done little to raise national concern.

Sound information about nutrition, obesity, fitness, avoidance of injury, exercise prescription, and a programmatic approach to wellness is readily available. The problem is not a lack of valid data, but of finding a way to integrate this information into daily life. All too often studies and educational efforts are directed to the already committed or limited to informing only other professionals. The physician as a fitness motivator should closely examine what those in the communication sciences can teach about education strategies.

Parents as Motivators

Every study on the influence of parents on a child's activity patterns has clearly demonstrated the significance of the parent in establishing the child's fitness ethic. The 1987 National Child and Youth Fitness Study II examined almost 5,000 parents in 19 states.[3] It showed that physical activity patterns had a significant impact on cardiorespiratory endurance and body conditioning. It also found that children's activity habits were most influenced by school physical education, out-of-school activities, and parental activity habits. These parents proved to be poor models of fitness or activity. Fewer than 30% of parents with 7- to 10-year-old children participated in any regular physical activity. About 50% of these parents never participated in any form of vigorous exercise. Those who exercised did so an average of less than once a week.

Gender stereotyping also has a great effect on female participation in physical activity. With the advent of Title IX and increased numbers of women in intercollegiate and interscholastic sports, physicians must act as resources about gender issues in sports. The significance of the parental role is an almost universal finding in examinations of the motivation and character make-up of elite female athletes.[4] More than 90% of these elite women were raised in a two-parent family setting.[5] During interviews, they said their fathers had generated a social and psychological milieu in which they felt free to become competitive athletes. They shared their father's masculine world in both recreation and sports. Their fathers and mothers shared androgynous attitudes and values. Current data continue to show that females with a positive sports ethic have experienced a more gender-free cultural environment. Thus, they are better able to defend themselves against negative gender stereotyping. Women who have maintained a fitness and exercise lifestyle beyond 40 years of age report that their mothers, also active participants, were a primary source of motivation. Thus, an increased level of parental participation, providing models for children to emulate, would be a strong motivating force.

A number of socioeconomic and cultural factors contribute to the lower sports participation by females and the gradual attrition that occurs between the ages of 6 and 16 years. According to studies, the critical drop-out rate correlates with the onset of adolescence, at about 12 years of age.[6] Social class and education also contribute to the negative curve of participation in athletics by females. When making presentations to the general public, physicians can provide an important service by relieving parents of their anxieties about their daughter's participation in athletics. Many parents wonder about the effects of sport participation on femininity, growth, maturation, and retention of feminine values and attitudes. Many believe that intense commitment to fitness or sports has a deleterious effect on physiologic functioning. Other parents, especially those with less education, are concerned that competitive sport participation will reduce their daughter's ability to form a heterosexual bond.

It is important to enlighten parents about endocrinologic, physiologic, and morphologic issues related to fitness. This can help relieve their anxieties and dispel their false beliefs and prejudices about the long-range effects of exercise and competitive sports on their daughters.

Educating the Parent-Coach

Those adults who give of their time as trainers may be the most effective agents of change. These volunteers demonstrate a level of motivation that distinguishes them from parents in general. Nonetheless, few communities have set standards or offer training to equip them for such responsible roles.

In 1972 Canada first addressed this problem as a national concern. The Interprovincial Council of Sport and Recreation began developing a model training program for all Canadian sports. Coaches, teachers, and psychologists met, held discussions, and exchanged ideas about the problem of untrained citizen-coaches. Through the efforts of the Coaching Association of Canada, national and provincial sports governing bodies designed technical training courses for sport, with guidelines and national training standards for coaches. Most importantly, they developed practical schedules for on-the-job training, where theories and principles could be applied and learned. In 1974 the first formal courses of the National Coaching Certificate program were offered.[7]

The Canadian effectiveness-training program is designed to meet three competency levels. Level I is directed to local or school coaches who work with 6- to 16-year-old athletes. Coaches with Levels II or III certification are qualified to coach any age group. The following is an example of the content of Levels I and II training.

Goals of Level I Training
1. Outline the social responsibilities of a coach's role.
2. List the important effects the coach has on athletes.
3. Select activities that foster fun and participation.
4. Practice basic communication skills.
5. Outline basic principles about how the body works and grows.
6. Analyze simple skills, detect errors, and know how to correct them according to movement principles.
7. Detect and correct unsafe playing conditions.
8. Practice the principles of effective teaching.
9. Plan sound practices.

Goals of Level II Training
1. Improve coaching leadership skills, especially in the areas of interpersonal communication, goal-setting, and role influence.
2. Outline the motivational needs of athletes and apply appropriate motivational principles.
3. Apply appropriate learning principles for skill performance based on sound teaching methods.
4. Describe soft-tissue injuries and apply emergency care in a variety of emergency situations.
5. Detect, analyze, and correct basic mechanical errors in skill performance.
6. Train athletes using sound physiologic principles.
7. Plan a seasonal program appropriate to goals, skill level, age, motivation, and needs of the athlete or team.

Level III training is designed to develop the skills of those who work with elite, national, Olympic, or professional athletes. The course content and instruction offered at Level III approach that of graduate university training. Formal written and oral examinations are required at each training level and certification is granted only to those who meet these criteria.

The Canadian certification program follows an East European training model. In the preface to the Level I manual, G.R. Gowan, Chairman, NCCC, states a training program philosophy that identifies the most worthy values and goals for all teaching professionals.

"I hope it is obvious that there is no such thing as mass participation v. excellence. They are inseparable! The more people we have involved in sport and the more skillful we become at designing programs which are appropriate to their talents and interests, the more opportunities there will be for people to achieve excellence, an excellence which is a very personal thing. The more we understand as coaches, the more we will be able to help thousands of boys and girls and men and women to derive satisfaction from their involvement in sport."

Creating Child-Centered Fitness Activities

The most frequently neglected training area has been an awareness of the child's psychosocial needs. Studies on children's motivation within organized sport programs suggest an interaction of specific psychosocial incentives. Although the priority of these incentives varies slightly, it is possible to identify the primary incentives. Children participate in sports to have fun, to become accepted members of the group, to measure their performance against those of other members of the group, to improve skills and performance, to enjoy freedom of physical expression, and to experience success, to be better than others.

Much has been written about using a child's intrinsic motivation and defining success as the process of learning and developing rather than simply winning. When children rank their reasons for participating, winning is near the end of the list.[8,9] There is a need for a values reorientation within our society, as evidenced by the negative adult behaviors associated with youth sports. Certainly the pediatrician must take a leading role as an educator and assume responsibility for creating a child-centered recreational and sports world. The primary factor behind the significant values shift in Canada that resulted in the creation of the certification program was the serious moral deterioration in youth hockey. Disgraceful behavior in highly organized and competitive youth programs forced educators, social scientists, coaches, and mental hygienists to reexamine the goals of sports participation. In the United States, there have been some areas of self-examination, but no regional, district, or national examination of the goals and aims of youth sport.

Medically and Psychologically Underserved Areas

There are particular psychosocial dangers for those select children who exhibit unusual motor gifts. These children will be in elite training programs and have above-average potential for athletic success. In figure skating, gymnastics, swimming, tennis, and other glamour sports, parents seem to have no compunction about placing 6-year-old children in highly structured programs. By the time these children are 10 to 12 years old, they may train four to six hours a day, six days a week. The competitive pressure imposed on those who attain district, regional, or national status has a compelling effect on their emotional adjustment. Those in sports medicine must take a responsible and active part as counselors for the welfare of these young elite athletes.

Inevitably, there will be emotional and social costs for which the child athlete is totally unprepared. Achievement, success, and recognition can create emotional burdens beyond the capacity of even the most emotionally mature child. These elite children should have the opportunity to sit with a professional and review all the negative factors associated with success. Children should be able to anticipate how they will confront these negatives. Such a review will reduce stress and enable them to practice effective coping strategies.

A vital concern is the danger that such children will become one-dimensional personalities. These children can establish their self-worth or self-esteem only through the expression of a single attribute or talent. They often have no other way of expressing themselves that enables them to feel that they are valued or worthy persons. Their egos are supported solely by success in the single domain of athletic achievement. The inherent danger of this is apparent, but the subtle form it takes is often masked by objective success. Parents, coaches, fans, and the community are so focused on accomplishment that other social and psychological needs remain unanswered.[10]

Educators must also examine the complex emotional and social issues associated with termination experiences within sports. National heroes or professional celebrities are not the only ones who experience sudden termination beyond their control. The same trauma can happen to the child athlete, if termination comes because of injury, maturational differences, motor competence, family decisions, or the capricious nature of a coach's judgment. In these cases, the child is unable to control what is happening. Children as young as 12 years old can exhibit symptoms of depression because injury or maturational changes prevent them from meeting competitive standards. Children and adults may move through the same stages of emotional crisis that characterize profound grief reaction.[11,12] The pediatrician can be a referral agent and provide these children with access to treatment for termination crises.

The Fitness, Recreational, and Sports Needs of the Disabled

The last decade has seen an explosion of interest in the value of fitness and sport for children with physical and mental limitations. An important catalyst for this interest has been the published investigations of the physical, social, and psychological factors associated with elite disabled competition. The elite wheelchair athletes in national, international, and Olympic competition have provided a data base from which to speculate about the value of such programs for all physically disadvantaged persons. Although these studies are limited in number and restricted in terms of ability, their findings have generated enthusiasm about the potential value of sports for the physically disadvantaged in general.

Studies have found that wheelchair athletes in national and international events are indistinguishable from elite able-bodied athletes. Personality structure, emotional make-up, and motivation for retaining positive athletic values are strikingly similar.[13,14] Standardized psychological measures of emotional characteristics and intrinsic motivational factors suggest the only difference is the level of physical limitation. When elite wheelchair athletes are compared with national Olympic-level competitors in such sports as wrestling, gymnastics, rowing, and basketball, the psychometric profiles of the able-bodied and the disabled athletes are almost identical.[15,16]

Investigations of the motivational forces that account for such a dedicated commitment to recreation and sport provide a powerful educational argument. They indicate that disabled and able-bodied athletes are expressing identical needs.[16] These factors may be categorized as Ego Incentives, Task Incentives, Social Incentives, Socialization Incentives, Fitness Incentives, and Self-Measurement Incentives. Here is how disabled athletes rank the needs met by participation in sports.

Rank Order of Incentives for Wheelchair Athletes

1. It offers me an opportunity to improve my level of health and fitness.
2. It offers me an opportunity to improve my ability.
3. I like to win.
4. I enjoy the excitement of the game.
5. I enjoy the team interaction.
6. It gives me a chance to perform game skills.
7. It gives me a chance to be with friends.
8. It offers me the chance to make new acquaintances.
9. It offers me a chance to compare my skills with others.
10. It offers me the opportunity to prove that I can compete against others successfully.
11. It gives me a chance to test myself against my own ideals.
12. It offers me a chance to travel.
13. I derive joy from the physical feeling of the experience.
14. It provides me with the opportunity for emotional release.
15. It offers me the opportunity to use good equipment.
16. It offers me a chance to gain recognition.
17. It enables me to feel wanted and needed by others.
18. It pleases others who are close to me.

Age, gender, and even limited physical capacity seem to have little bearing on the level of motivation or on the quality of these incentives. Only the incentive value of new or more advanced equipment actually distinguishes these wheelchair athletes from athletes in general.

Is more empirical data on social, psychological, and motivating needs necessary before these expressed incentives become the basis for program development and education? The ideal recreation, activity, or sports environment would meet these basic human incentives and the needs of every child from age 4 through early adulthood.

The Parent, the Child, and the Role of the Coach

Health educators face a complex and sensitive responsibility in establishing and maintaining effective communication among child, coach, and parent. It is difficult to know how many children are actively participating in organized youth programs. As youth sports become more highly structured and as parents become more involved in the child's activities, problems become more complex. The issues of transportation, expense, and parental involvement in supporting or managing the activity have forced increased interactions among child, coach, and parent.

The educator must provide guidelines to enable parents to reinforce those things that are most valuable for their child's development. For the child's growth and development, the health educator must define appropriate parental behavior and set boundaries on parental conduct. This issue is also important to coaches. An entire clinic could be devoted to educating parents, and a second to teaching coaches how to deal effectively with parents. In any given program, there will be a broad range of parenting styles. Some parents are so overidentified with their child's experiences that they cannot communicate in an objective manner. Others feel their total responsibility is simply to bring the child to the event. Within this range is every level of communication problem.

An important aspect of parenting is living vicariously through the experiences of one's child. The problems arise when the parent loses perspective on the boundary between parent and child. Issues become clouded when the parents' strong or inappropriate feelings distort their perceptions of what is happening in the life of their child. Often, the traumas of the child athlete reflect parental violation of the required emotional boundaries. The pediatrician can render an important service by conducting preseason parent-education sessions. Professionals in the behavior sciences can address the appropriate role of the parent in the child's athletic life, and provide insights on how to create a better mental and social environment for the child.

These sessions should include the coaching staff. Coaches could outline their philosophies and goals as teachers, describe the ideal parent-coach relationship, and outline acceptable child behavior. The coach should have the opportunity to outline a code of conduct for parents and children, and spell out the steps taken when code violations occur. The pediatrician should encourage a dialogue that leads to a parent-coach consensus on expected conduct, spelled out in a formal contract between coach and parent. This can help reinforce parental conduct and responsibility when crises arise or communication has eroded.

Some issues occur frequently within high-level competitive youth sports programs. These include the extent to which parents are willing to subordinate their needs to the needs of their children, parents who feel strongly that their child is not receiving the same level of attention as others, parents who feel that there is too great a training load on their child, parents who feel their rights are being violated because the coach wishes to maintain a privileged communication relationship with the child, parents who rebel when the coach suggests that performance problems are related to external causes, parents who refuse to abide by a code of conduct at events, and parents who refuse to accept the coach's side of any issue when coach-athlete communication has broken down.

Hundreds of other situations could be listed but these are enough to make an important point: prevention by anticipation is the best strategy. Collaborative acceptance of a structured outline of expectations will reduce miscommunication and possible conflict.

References

1. Ross JG, Gilbert GG: The National Children and Youth Fitness Study: A Summary of Findings, J Phys Educ Recreat Dance 1987;58:50-96.
2. Anderson C: Childhood fitness: The importance of parents. *The Melpomene Journal*, Spring 1988.
3. The National Children and Youth Fitness Study, II. J. Phys Educ Recreat Dance 1987;58:50-96.
4. Ogilvie BC: Women who dared to succeed in sports. In Knight J, Slovendo R (eds): Psychological motivation in play and sports, Springfield, IL, Charles C. Thomas, 1969, pp 149-156.
5. Pollock JC, Bailey JG: Miller Lite Report on Women in Sport, New World Decisions Ltd, Iselin, New Jersey, December 1985.
6. The Wilson Report: Daughter's reasons for discontinuing sport participation. Diagnostic Research, Inc, Los Angeles, CA.
7. National Coaching Association Certification Council: Coaching Association of Canada, 333 River Road Ottawa, Canada, K1L 8B9, 1979.
8. Ogilvie BC: The orthopaedist's role in children's sports. *Orthop Clin No Amer* 1983;14:361-372.
9. Ogilvie BC: The child and adolescent in sports: A Psychological profile, in Birrer RB (ed): *Sports Medicine for the Primary Care Physician.* Norwalk, Appleton-Century-Crofts, 1984, ch 28.
10. Ogilvie BC: Counseling patients with career-ending injuries, in Feagin J (ed): *The Crucial Ligaments: The Diagnosis and Treatment of Ligamentous Injuries About the Knee.* Philadelphia, JB Lippincott, 1987, pp 357-366.
11. Ogilvie BC: The case for career termination counseling, in Williams J (ed): *Personal Growth to Peak Performance.* Mountain View, California Mayfield Publishing, 1986, pp 365-387.
12. Ogilvie BC: Counseling for career termination, in May JR, Asken MJ (eds): *Sports Psychology: The Psychological Health of the Athlete.* New York, PMA Publishing, 1987, pp 213-230.
13. Sherrill C, Rainbolt W: Self-actualization of male able-bodied and elite cerebral palsy athletes. *Adapt Phys Educ Quart* 1988;5.
14. Brasile FD: The psychological factors that influence participation in wheelchair basketball. *Palaestra* 1988;4:16-19.
15. Henchen K, Horvat M, French R: A visual comparison of psychological profiles between able-bodied and wheelchair athletes. *Adapt Phys Active Quarterly* 1984;1,2:pp118-124.
16. Cooper S, Shreill C, Marshall D: Attitudes towards physical activities of elite cerebral palsy athletes. *Adapt Phys Activities Quarterly.* (In Press)

Chapter 13

The Pediatric Athlete and Role Modeling

Richard H. Gross, MD

Introduction

A role model should be a person whose life is an example for imitation. How children select role models is poorly understood. Although role models are important for today's young athletes, the literature on this subject is "diffuse" according to Rainer Martens.[1] Role models are ephemeral and subject to change without notice. They are a paradigm of the time, and the spirit and tone of the time determines the nature and character of the role model.

Historical Perspective

Role models for the young athlete did not become a subject for study until this century. Sport for children in the past either was not a factor or had quite a different tenor. Phillipe Aries' exhaustive study[2] of childhood through the centuries notes that childhood had no place in the medieval world. Paintings from that time depict that "any gathering for the purpose of work, relaxation, or sport brought together both children and adults."[2] The 1556 French publication, *Le Grande Proprietaire de toutes choses* described the stages of life, saying "there are only three in French, to wit, childhood, youth, and old age."[2] One was a child while dependent, then a youth, until one became physically weakened, then came old age. There were no children's sports, for after age 3 or 4, children and adults played the same games.

Before the sixteenth century, sport was not considered as a vehicle for moral training, and young children of 5 or 6 could gamble or attend cockfights, plays, and dances. Two distinctions became prominent about this time—childhood from adulthood, and lower from upper class. Churchmen and moralists saw children as fragile creatures who needed safeguarding and moral training.

School for children began in the fifteenth century, and pupils were separated by ability, not age. Schools were rough places and mutinies by students were common, especially in England.[2] To counter these mutinies, schoolmasters employed strict discipline and humiliation. Finally, separate schools for the wealthy were begun with emphasis on the classics.

In these times, before child labor laws, lower-class children worked, married, and had children.[3] Marriage in the American colonies commonly took place between children in their early teens. At the time of the Revolution, boys became landowners and militiamen at 16.[4]

The Industrial Revolution of the nineteenth century fostered the development of overcrowded urban areas and miserable childhoods for the working class. Few working-class children had more than two or three years of school. Until the late nineteenth century, sports had almost no place in the young person's life. At an early age children assumed adult behaviors and responsibilities. There was no need for sport or fitness role models.

Role Modeling in the Twentieth Century

In the late nineteenth century, the Christian Socialist movement, with its goal of Muscular Christianity, assumed prominence.[5,6] Schools broadened their curriculum by introducing science, modern history, foreign languages, and stressing character building. The major vehicle for moral training was team sports that promoted the spirit of "manliness." The Christian Socialist movement found fertile ground in America, especially in the eastern aristocracy. Thomas Wentworth Higginson, a Harvard Divinity School graduate, wrote a number of books for boys on behavior. They promoted patriotism and self-control and advised boys to display little affection and to curtail sexual appetites through devotion to wholesome, rugged activity. Tenets of Muscular Christianity can be found in Teddy Roosevelt's advice: "In life, as in a football game, the principle to follow is: hit the line hard, don't foul, and don't shirk, but hit the line hard!" A disciple of this approach was Luther Halsey Gulick, who became involved with the YMCA in 1887.[5] He was an indefatigable worker and organized a competitive program at the YMCA training school despite formidable opposition. In 1903, he became the first Director of Physical Training in the public schools of New York. Youth sports could only thrive in a relatively urban environment, where there were enough children to form competitive teams.

Early twentieth-century writings portray the athlete in glowing terms.[7] The dominant philosophy was that a sound mind and body went hand in hand. The sexes were separated, and youth sports were for boys only.

Professional sports provided heroes and role models, including Red Grange, Babe Ruth, Lou Gehrig, Joe DiMaggio, Jack Dempsey, Helen Wills, and many more.

In the 1960s heroes in the traditional sense disappeared. Sports writing changed, and private lives as well as public performance were subject to scrutiny. Jim Bouton turned the baseball world upside down with *Ball Four*, published in 1970.[8] Bouton discussed a newsletter published by Lindy McDaniel of the Yankees.

> One of the first I got from him—and all the players receive them—was a complete four-page explanation of why the Church of Christ was the only true church. The philosophy here is that religion is the reason an athlete is good at what he does. . . . So I've been tempted sometimes to say into a microphone that I feel I won tonight because I don't believe in God. I mean, just for the sake of balance, to let the kids know that belief in a deity of "Pitching for the Master" is not one of the criteria for major league success. But I guess I never will.[8]

In *The Boz*, the association between moral life and sports disappeared completely. According to Brian Bosworth,

> I also find it no problem to cheat in the NFL, partly because the refs are so old and crawling with barnacles. The best time is when the clock is winding down. . . . That's a great time, if you're in a pile, to twist someone's head or put your finger in his earhole and try to rearrange his hearing.[9]

Sport is a very complicated business. Records that seemed impossible a generation ago are now commonplace. Athletes are bigger and stronger, and they train harder. But what does all this mean to the young athlete? Who are his or her role models? What forces will mold the characters of new role models?

Role models are necessary, particularly accessible, local role models. Sooner or later, youths who participate in sports will have to learn how to handle failure. Pat Conroy, in *The Great Santini*, says

> Sports shows you your limits. Sports teaches humility. Sooner or later the athlete becomes humble no matter how good he is. But he plays until he has reached as high as he can.[10]

Who would be a better teacher than an older child who has already learned these lessons? Older children are the most underrecognized and underused source of role models[11] for the overwhelming majority of young athletes who must still come to grips with the consequences of failure and humility. Youth coaches can also be important role models. Pat Conroy gives an excellent description of a coach.[12]

> A coach occupies a high place in a boy's life. . . . If they are lucky, good coaches can become the perfect unobtainable father that young boys dream about and rarely find in their own homes. . . . Good coaches shape and exhort and urge. . . . Through sports a coach can offer a boy a secret way to sneak upon the mystery that is manhood.

Rainer Martens' American Coaching Effectiveness Program is an example of an endeavor in this direction.[13] Training coaches to meet these expectations is necessary.

A fundamental problem with sport role models is that the perspective has changed drastically in the last 50 years. For young people, sports should be a challenge to do their best. The emphasis should not be to win at all costs, as it seems in college and professional sports. The healthy, fit individual should be the role model, and should maintain an active lifestyle *all his or her life* as part of a balanced approach.

There is no hard science about role models, only observations and opinions. Times and role models will undoubtedly continue to change. Understanding them in perspective is the critical first step.

Bibliography

1. Martens R: *Personal Communication.* 1988.
2. Aries P: *Centuries of Childhood: A Social History of Family Life.* New York, Vintage Books, 1962.
3. Kotker N (ed): *The Horizon Book of the Elizabethan World.* New York, American Heritage Publishing, 1967.
4. Earle AM: *Child Life in Colonial Days.* New York, Macmillan, 1899.
5. Wiggins DK: A History of Organized Play and Highly Competitive Sport for American Children in Gould D, Weiss M (eds). *Advances in Pediatric Sport Sciences* vol 2. Champaign, Human Kinetics, 1987.
6. Altick RD: *Victorian People and Ideas.* New York, London, WW Norton, 1973.
7. Atkinson L, Lake A: *Famous Athletes of Today.* Boston, LC Page and Co, 1932.
8. Bouton J: *Ball Four.* New York, Dell, 1970.
9. Bosworth B, Reilly R: *The Boz: Confessions of a Modern Anti-Hero.* New York, Doubleday, 1988.
10. Conroy P: *The Great Santini.* New York, Bantam, 1977.
11. Holt J: *How Children Learn.* New York, Dell, 1967.
12. Conroy P: *The Prince of Tides.* New York, Bantam, 1986.
13. Martens R, Christina RW, Harvey JS, et al: *Coaching Young Athletes.* Champaign, Human Kinetics, 1981.

Chapter 14

Fitness and the School Curriculum

William A. Grana, MD

Introduction

The first National Children and Youth Fitness Study (NCYFS I) examined children ten to 17 years old. Its results were extended in the second National Children and Youth Fitness Study (NCYFS II) to determine the role and effects of health-related fitness in a younger age group, kindergarten to grade 4.[1] This chapter will examine some of the results of this second study, the fitness habits of children, the factors affecting fitness and the school-age child, the impact of fitness programs, and some prototype elementary health-related fitness programs.

Physical Fitness and the Schoolchild

For young children, fitness promotes health and well-being and can contribute to academic achievement by improving the overall quality of life. Young children are highly interested in fitness activities, but by the time they are juniors and seniors in high school, most no longer participate in any fitness programs. Educating young children to the value of fitness will improve their chances of developing good health habits for adult life.

The physical-fitness habits of young children have worsened since the 1960s.[2] Skin-fold testing shows changes in body composition. Lean body mass is decreasing and body fat is increasing. Sit-and-reach tests also show flexibility is decreasing.[1]

Where Does Fitness Activity Occur?

The schools have a pivotal role in determining the exercise habits of children.[3] In grades 1 to 4, 97% of children are enrolled in physical education. In addition, extracurricular activities help make the transition from movement activities to sports in this age group.[1] It is important that physical fitness programs for school-age children embrace a wide range of activities that include, but are not limited to, competitive sports if the goal of lifetime fitness is achieved.[4]

Fitness begins at home, according to 30% of parents of children in grades 1 to 4, and these 30% participate in vigorous fitness activities. But more than 50% of parents engage in no vigorous fitness activity at all.[1] On the average, parents spend less than one day a week in vigorous physical activity. At the same time, their children spend two hours per weekday and 3.5 hours per weekend day watching television. Finally, both parents and teachers encourage boys to participate in physical activity more than they do girls.[1]

Community organizations, such as parks and recreation programs, Little Leagues, church programs, YMCA and YWCA programs, and scouting organizations, play a significant role in promoting health-related fitness. Of children in grades 1 through 4, 85% participate in such programs. However, these programs emphasize competitive sports and exclude health-related fitness activities. In addition, twice as many boys participate as girls.[1]

This confirms that the role of the school is key in educating and encouraging participation in health-related fitness programs. Children are first exposed to organized fitness and sports through school and can develop the habit of regular participation in physical activity.[5]

What Determines Fitness in School?

A number of variable factors affect school fitness programs. While 97% of schoolchildren participate, they fall into two distinct groups: those who participate on a daily basis (36% of the children studied), and those who participate one day or less per week (37% of the children studied). Although 80% of the children participate in programs with a physical education specialist, only a third of these specialists are certified. In addition, only 40% of the children have special facilities, and more than half participate in the schoolyard without the benefit of special equipment. Schools tend not to invest in physical education facilities or specialists.[1]

Fitness testing is an integral part of a fitness program.[6] Since elementary schools have not adopted health-related fitness testing on a broad basis, the value of their physical education programs cannot be assessed.[1] Many teachers do not like to give fitness tests or do not have the training necessary to administer the tests.[1] Since performance is not recognized, children will not realize the importance of participating in a fitness program. For programs to succeed, the amount of time, the number of qualified instructors, and the available facilities must be improved. These factors are not under teachers' control.[4,1]

On the other hand, teachers can work within their current programs and develop objectives to promote health-related fitness. They can select age-appropriate activities for the children, they can make the most of the time and the facilities that are available to them, and they can adopt fitness testing to encourage regular exercise and those activities which promote a healthy lifestyle.[1]

Impact of Fitness

Fitness testing indicates that those children who perform well in the walk/run participate in more fitness activities than other children. They watch less television and are considered more physically active by their parents and teachers. Their parents are also more active.[1] The majority of adults feel that physical education is important for children, and 89% of parents disapprove of substituting other courses for physical education. In addition, 86% believe the primary concern of a school's physical education program should be physical fitness. When asked about content, 99% of parents said these programs should focus on determining the best way to exercise and the importance of exercise for children. Parents felt that endurance-type physical fitness activities were the most important, followed by individual sports, team sports, and recreational games. However, the emphasis in school programs remains on competitive sports, often to the exclusion of health-related fitness activities.[1]

The goals of physical fitness programs should be to maintain high-quality health, to improve fitness and physiologic function, to develop psychomotor performance skills, to develop personal health and fitness habits, and to integrate them into a positive lifestyle and interaction with others.[1,5,6]

Prototype Elementary School Health-Related Fitness Program

Currently there are state-mandated requirements in physical education in 41 states, but 60% of those programs require less than 300 hours of physical education for kindergarten through 12th grade. Less than 3% of the total instructional time for educational activities is spent on physical education.

In Europe, there is a greater emphasis on physical fitness. For example, in the German Democratic Republic, the Education Act makes physical education compulsory in all educational institutions. Physical education sessions must be held twice a week in grades 1 to 3 with similar or increasing demands in advanced grades. In addition, after-school and vacation activities supplement and coordinate with school activities. For example, swimmers can participate in groups and achievement-recognition programs emphasizing participation, not competition. The East Germans believe this is the reason for the high level of fitness in the population as a whole. Their program could serve as a prototype for the United States.[7]

In the 41 states that mandate health-related fitness activity, programs vary greatly. Although considerable thought may be given to establishing the purpose, objectives, and goals of these programs, the end result may not be the most desirable result. Most programs confirm the need to integrate cognitive and psychomotor areas through health-related fitness activities and to use these activities in developing the total personality of the child, including moral and ethical qualities. Few recognize the corollary: that competitive sports, with the primary emphasis on winning, is only a small part of such fitness activities, and developing good health habits requires more than interscholastic athletic programs.[4,6,8]

Oklahoma is one of nine states without a mandate for health-related fitness. There is no set curriculum for physical education. Some communities have physical education specialists certified for kindergarten through 12th grade; others specify kindergarten through sixth grade. Special facilities may not be available in many areas, so physical education takes place in the cafeteria or on the school grounds.

A constant dichotomy exists between the health-related fitness approach and the competitive-sports approach to physical education for children. If the physical education specialist is mainly interested in coaching, there will be a rapid transition to emphasizing competitive sports. This approach may actually turn children away from fitness activities rather than encourage participation. To avoid this problem, coaches must be very sensitive to the needs of young children and allow them to explore a full range of activities.

In Edmond, Oklahoma, children in kindergarten through fourth grade have two 30-minute sessions of physical education and one 30-minute health program per week. These may or may not be integrated depending on the individual teacher. In addition, fitness activities also depend on the individual teacher's interests.

Summary

Health-related fitness programs need to integrate the cognitive and psychomotor areas to develop the whole person. Sports focus on psychomotor abilities, but do not emphasize good health habits for life. Although 41 of 50 states have mandates for health-related fitness activities, a national survey shows that today's children are less fit than children were 20 years ago. There is a crisis in the public schools about the direction and value of health-related fitness programs in the curriculum.

References

1. The National Children and Youth Fitness Study II: *J of Phys Ed Rec and Dance* 1987;58:50-95.
2. US Department of Health and Human Services: *Promoting Health/Preventing Disease: Objectives for the Nation.* Washington, DC. Government Printing Office, 1980.
3. Bennett WJ: *First Lessons: A Report on Elementary Education in America.* Washington, DC. Government Printing Office, 1986.

4. Coach the Coaches. *NEA TODAY* September 1988;7(1):2.

5. Powell KE, Spain KG, Christenson GM, Mollenkamp MP: The status of the 1990 objectives for physical fitness and exercise. *Public Health Reports* 1986; 101(1):15-20.

6. *A Guide to Curriculum Development in Physical Education.* Connecticut State Board of Education, Hartford, 1981.

7. Marschner P: Sports education in the German Democratic Republic. *Prospects* 1976;6:1.

8. Mitchell MF, Earls RF: A profile of state requirements. *The Physical Educator* Fall 1987;44(3):337-43.

Chapter 15

The Structure of Youth and Amateur Sports in the United States

J. Andy Sullivan, MD
Don E. Porter, MD

Introduction

Sports are tests of skill undertaken primarily for the diversion of those who participate in or observe them. The origins of most sports remain obscure. Children, when given the opportunity, organize games that measure their skills against each other. The rules they establish tend to allow fair competition, high scoring, and full participation.[1]

In the past 100 years, there has been a tremendous growth in the number of organizations supporting youth and amateur sports. These organizations should provide stability to meet the goals of their members.[2,3] If children participate in games primarily for pleasure or fun, the organization should be structured to meet that need. This chapter reviews the history and current structure of youth sports organizations and surveys how well these organizations are meeting their goals. A more complete history of the development of youth sports is given in "A History of Organized Play and Highly Competitive Sport for American Children" by David K. Wiggins.[4]

History of Youth Sports

Youth sports organizations first appeared in the latter part of the 1800's. The Young Men's Christian Association was founded by evangelical Protestants in England in 1851. In the early decades of the twentieth century, Boys' Clubs and the Boy Scouts also provided recreational opportunities in organized sports. The early impetus for these groups came largely from a group known as the Crusade for Muscular Christianity, who advocated a return to the Greek ideal of the harmonious development of the mind, body, and spirit. Fitness, outdoor activities, and sports were ways of achieving this end.

The public school system also offered structured sport opportunities for children. The New York Board of Education program gave every child the opportunity to participate in sport, based on the individual's ability. Although girls could participate in this early program, their involvement was restricted.

Chicago's South Park District developed the first city playgrounds in 1903. Three years later, the Playground Association of America was founded, and has remained a primary advocate for the right of children to play. In the 1920s and 1930s, programs began to move out of the school and into the private sector. This movement of sport to volunteer organizations coincided with a growing concern by educators that sports were overemphasized in schools and were potentially detrimental. Volunteer youth organizations evolved to support their particular areas of interest. Many of the organizations founded during this period are still in existence today, such as Pop Warner football and Little League baseball. Other associations were started by Olympic groups, colleges, businesses, churches, and other not-for-profit groups.

Girls participated in sports in these early organizations, but their opportunities were, and still are, limited. Despite legislation mandating equal opportunities, discrimination often results in less participation from girls. Even in organizations that seem not to discriminate, subtle differences can lead to greater participation by males than by females.

In 1979, the National Council of Youth Sports Directors (NCYSD) and the North American Youth Sport Institute (NAYSI) brought together many diverse organizations. NAYSI conducts workshops and clinics and sponsors youth sport-related research programs.

In addition to individual youth-sports organizations, a number of peripheral organizations support youth sports.[5] One example is the American Coaching Effectiveness Program started by Brian J. Craddy and Ranier Martens. A growing number of sports psychologists are helping promote more effective leadership for sports organizations.

Podilchak described the development of youth-sports structures in an article analyzing two levels of competition: house leagues and selective leagues.[6] He states that youth-sports organizations achieve legitimacy by following certain societal norms and by organizing themselves in much the same manner as businesses and governing bodies. By doing so they hope to achieve lobbying power to support children's sports. House leagues operate on a local level to organize children, provide competition, and emphasize fun and enjoyment for players. Selective leagues establish a tryout process based on a display of skills, involve a geographically wider competitive program, and emphasize skill and performance.

Selective leagues have higher organizational bodies and connections to higher-level sports organizations. House leagues, with a neighborhood emphasis, develop few interorganizational links. House leagues measure performance by participation. In selective leagues performance is measured by proficiency.

Podilchak also examined resource dependency or the flow of resources. To succeed, an organization needs human resources, facilities, and sufficient capital to operate. All youth sports depend to a greater or lesser extent on volunteers for these resources. As youth organizations grow, their resource needs eventually exceed the ability of volunteers to provide them. At that point money is needed to hire an administrative staff.

Facilities must be obtained and this may require the cooperation of other sports or other public bodies. Ties can be established between organizations that have similar goals (football and soccer join together to obtain new playing fields) or between organizations to reach a broader area and larger constituency (two soccer clubs join together to obtain a new complex).

Stable organizations can approach benefactors and ask for program support, donations of land or facilities, and other resources. Podilchak explained that house leagues have difficulty surviving because they lack access to resources or power. He also suggested that for sports to develop stability and ensure survival, there must be a shift to more selective leagues. With this shift, sport leagues are able to ensure their survival and obtain access to facilities and resources.

Basically, sports programs are developed by adults who have children interested in playing. Initially these programs are fairly small and frequently emphasize participation. Eventually, some participants show greater levels of skill than their peers. These individuals must be challenged or they will become bored. Similarly, less-skilled individuals will become bored if they have to sit on the bench and watch the talented players perform. A good youth-sports organization can provide for both types of players.

Sports organizations have evolved over the last 100 years as a way to involve children in sports.[1,7] Although an organizational structure is necessary, do these organizations meet the goals of the participants? For example, the organizational structure of the Soviet youth-sport system is rigidly controlled from Moscow.[8,9] Its principal goal is to maintain Soviet dominance in international competitions such as the Olympics. In the United States, adults have suggested varied goals for youth sports,[2,3,10,11] such as (1) diversion and the development of fitness habits that can carry over into adult life, (2) relief of anxiety, (3) physical fitness, and (4) development of leadership skills and teamwork abilities.

Survey Results

To determine the goals of youth-sports organizations, 23 organizations were surveyed. The questionnaire has no scientific validity, but it did obtain information about the structure of youth-sports organizations. Survey questions included: Do you follow the guidelines in the Athlete's Bill of Rights? (Outline 1) Are all children guaranteed a chance to participate? Do they have qualified supervision?

Ten organizations responded to the survey, representing the sports of baseball, gymnastics, hockey, soccer, swimming, field hockey, and football. In some sports, more than one organization responded. Each

Outline 1. Bill of Rights for Young Athletes
1. The right to participate in sports.
2. The right to participate on a level commensurate with each child's maturity and ability.
3. The right to have qualified adult leadership.
4. The right to play as a child and not as an adult.
5. The right of children to share in the leadership and decision-making of their sports participation.
6. The right to participate in safe and healthy environments.
7. The right to proper preparation for participation in sport.
8. The right to an equal opportunity to strive for success.
9. The right to be treated with dignity.
10. The right to have fun in sports.

organization's by-laws were reviewed to see if the goals were stated. The questionnaire asked whether the goals were followed.

All organizations encouraged the training of coaches and 20% provided clinics. Although all encouraged participation in the clinics, only 20% required it, so training is largely up to the individual. Training of officials was provided by 80% of the organizations.

Nearly all organizations provided various levels of participation. Recreational leagues were sponsored by 80% of the organizations, 90% provided all-star or select teams, and 80% had regional or national teams.

The question regarding participation generated some confusion. Roughly 60% of the respondents indicated that all participants were guaranteed a chance to play, but 80% also said that this varied at different levels of competition.

The young participants had some part in governing 60% of the organizations at the local and national level. Nearly all organizations (90%) had some affiliation or avenue for the participant who desired to be an Olympian. Most used age to determine the level of participation, but football and wrestling used size. All organizations had rules regarding fields or facilities.

A review of the by-laws showed that most of the organizations were in existence to "promote" that particular youth sport. Words such as "encourage," "enjoyment," "pleasure," or "for the fun of the kids" were rare.

Summary

In the United States, youth-sports structures have evolved to promote the individual sports and ensure their survival. As a result, there is more emphasis on individual skill and winning than on participation for fun. The number of children who ultimately play sports in college, the Olympics, or professional leagues is miniscule compared with the number of children who participate for fun. Youth-sports organizations must ultimately provide for both needs. This requires different levels of sophistication and the knowledge that elite athletes are a minority. Sports participation must be fun if it is to continue into adult life. Youth-sports organizations need to be aware of this important fact, and to reread the Athlete's Bill of Rights.[12]

Adolescent and high-school athletes must often make a choice to play school sports or continue at a recreational level.[7] Many drop out of athletics at this level. The structure of amateur athletics for this age group merges into adult organizations, which are discussed in the next section.

Structure of Amateur Sports

Amateur sports are organized under three organizations: the International Olympic Committee (IOC), the International Sports Federations, and the National Olympic Committees. Each has specific functions and responsibilities. This section outlines amateur sport functions and organizations in the United States.

International Olympic Committee

The IOC was created by the Congress of Paris on June 23, 1894 and entrusted with the control and development of the modern Olympic Games. The IOC is the final authority on all questions concerning the Olympic Games and the Olympic movement.

The IOC has four primary goals: (1) to encourage the organization and development of sports and sport competitions; (2) to inspire and lead sports within the Olympic ideal, thereby promoting and strengthening friendship between the athletes of all countries; (3) to ensure the regular celebration of the Olympic Games, and (4) to make the Olympic Games ever more worthy of their history and of the high ideals that inspired their revival by Baron Pierre de Coubertin and his associates.

International Sports Federations and National Governing Bodies

Each International Sports Federation is an autonomous organization, responsible for the international governance of its sport. Each federation conducts the events in its sports at the Olympic Games, and in other international competitions, in conjunction with the IOC and other National Olympic Committees.

Each federation establishes the eligibility rules for its sport. On occasion, one set of eligibility rules, approved by the IOC, is used in the Olympic Games while another set of rules is used in other international competitions.

Generally, a single federation governs each Olympic sport. However, speed skating and figure skating are both governed by the same federation, and the modern pentathlon and the biathlon are under a single federation.

For a sport to be added to the Olympic Games, the IOC must recognize the sports federation under the principles of the IOC's charter. Then, the federation must prove that the sport is "widely practiced," which means that national championships, world championships, and international competitions are held in at least 50 countries on three continents for men's sports and in 35 countries on three continents for women's sports. Only sports widely practiced by men and/or women in at least 25 countries on three continents may be included in the Olympic Winter Games.

Even if these requirements are met, however, the sport still may not become part of the Olympic Games. The 15 IOC-recognized federations whose sports are not in the Olympic Games (although some have been demonstration sports) include those for aeronautics, badminton, baseball, bowling, curling, karate, lawn bowling, orienteering, pelota basque (jai alai), racketball, roller skating, softball, sports acrobatics, squash, tae kwon do, and water skiing.

Each International Sports Federation recognizes a single National Governing Body in each country participating in the sport. Membership in the NGB must be open to all athletes in the country and to all national organizations concerned with promoting the sport. A national governing body is responsible for approving (sanctioning) competitions open to all athletes in its country. These competitions must then be conducted under the rules set by the governing body.

United States Olympic Committee

History   The US Olympic Committee (USOC), headquartered in Colorado Springs, is an organization of organizations. It is the central coordinating body for amateur sports in the United States, governing sports in the Olympic and Pan American Games, and those that want to be included in those games.

The USOC is recognized by the IOC as the sole agency in the United States responsible for training, entering, and underwriting the full expenses of the US teams in the Olympic and Pan American Games. The USOC also supports American cities that want to host the Winter or Summer Olympic Games or the Pan American Games. After reviewing all the candidates, the USOC votes on and endorses one city per event as the US bid city. The USOC also selects host cities for the US Olympic Festival and approves trial sites for the Olympic and Pan American Games.

Public Law 95-606 (The Amateur Sports Act) recognizes and regulates the USOC and its governance councils. It specifically names the USOC as the coordinating body in the United States for amateur activity directly relating to international amateur competitions, such as the

Olympic and Pan American Games. It also includes provisions for recognizing national governing bodies for the sports included in the Olympic and Pan American Games. Under this Act, the USOC is responsible for improving amateur athletics by encouraging developmental programs in various sports.

This public law not only protects the emblems of the IOC and the USOC but also gives the USOC exclusive rights to the words "Olympic" and "*Citius, Altius, Fortius*" (the Olympic motto) in the United States. It specifies that "recent or active" athletes must constitute at least 20% of the membership and voting power in all governance councils of the USOC. The law further states: "The Corporation shall be nonpolitical and, as an organization, shall not promote the candidacy of any person seeking public office."

Purpose and Goals   The USOC is dedicated to providing opportunities for American athletes of all ages and at all skill levels, and to preparing and training those athletes for the challenges of domestic competitions and the Olympic Games. The objects and purposes of the USOC include the following:

(1) To establish national goals for amateur athletic activities and encourage the attainment of those goals.

(2) To coordinate and develop amateur athletic activity in the United States directly relating to international competitions, and to foster productive working relationships among sports-related organizations.

(3) To exercise exclusive jurisdiction, either directly or through its constituent members of committees, over all matters pertaining to the participation and representation of the United States in the Olympic and Pan American Games and over the organization of the Olympic and Pan American Games when held in the United States.

(4) To obtain for the United States, whether directly or by delegation to the appropriate national (sports) governing body, the most competent amateur representation possible in each competition and event of the Olympic and Pan American Games.

(5) To promote and support amateur athletic activities involving the United States and foreign nations.

(6) To provide for the swift resolution of conflicts and disputes involving amateur athletes, national governing bodies or amateur sports organizations and to protect the opportunity of any amateur athlete, coach, trainer, manager, administrator, or official to participate in amateur athletic competitions.

(7) To foster the development of facilities and assist in making existing facilities available for use by amateur athletes.

(8) To encourage and support research, development, and dissemination of information in the areas of sports medicine, science, and safety.

(9) To encourage and provide assistance to amateur athletic activities for women, the handicapped, and athletes from racial or ethnic minorities.

The Structure of US Amateur Sports

Amateur sports in the United States are organized under the USOC, which serves as the central coordinating body in the administration, organization, and promotion of amateur athletic and sports competitions.

Each national governing body recognized by the USOC must, by law, administer and operate its sports under specific guidelines and procedures. The all-encompassing directive is "to develop interest and participation throughout the United States and be responsible to the persons and amateur sports organizations it represents."

National governing bodies must also "minimize scheduling conflicts with events, provide for sanctions to athletes and teams to compete outside the United States, encourage and support women's participation, support and encourage sports programs for the handicapped, provide for development in equipment design, coaching, officiating and performance, and encourage and support research, development and dissemination of information in sports medicine and sports safety."

The Amateur Sports Act provides a number of specifics to guide the national governing bodies. A complete copy of the Amateur Sports Act of 1978 can be obtained by requesting Public Law 95-606 of the 95th Congress.

References

1. Coakley JJ: Children and the Sports Socialization Process, in Gould and Weiss (eds). *Adv Pediatr Sport Sciences Vol II Behavioral Issues*. Human Kinetics, Champaign, IL.
2. Cleary B: National and Olympic Teams Should be Youth Goals, *US Hockey/Arena Biz* 1977;5(2):19-20.
3. Duda JL: Consider the Children: Meeting Participants' Goals in Youth Sports, *JOPERD* Aug, 1985;55-56.
4. Wiggins DK: A History of Organized Play and Highly Competitive Sport for American Children, in Gould and Weiss (eds). *Adv Pediatr Sport Sciences Vol II Behavioral Issues* ed. Human Kinetics, Champaign, IL.
5. Ferrel JM: Educating Youth Sport Coaches: Solutions to a National Dilemma. *YMCA Youth Sports Training Programs* American Alliance for Health, Physical Education and Recreation, 1982;83-88.
6. Podilchak W: Organizational Analysis of Youth Sports. *Int Review of Sport Sociology*, Warsaw, Poland, 1983;3:18.
7. Herrmann DE, Seefeldt V: What is the Future of Sports for High School-Age Youth?, *Athletic Purchasing and Facilities* 1982;6(10):14-18.
8. Jeffries SC: An Analysis of the Organizational Structure of Soviet Youth Sports System, in Redmond G (ed). *Sports and Politics*, Human Kinetics, Champaign, IL.
9. Svoboda B: Pedagogical Aspects of Youth Sports, *International Council of Sport Science and Physical Education Review*, 1985;8:16-24.
10. Brandt EN, McGinnis JM: National Children and Youth Fitness Study: Its Contribution to Our National Objectives, (editorial), *Public Health Reports*, Jan/Feb 1985;1-3.
11. Hilgers L: Stress Free Little League *Sports Illustrated*.
12. Shinnick P: Youth and Athlete's Rights, *ARENA*: The Institute for Sport and Social Analysis, May, 1982;6:40-42.

Appendix

Members of the USOC fall into five groups: The National Governing Bodies, National Multi-sports Organization, Affiliated Sports Organizations, State Olympic Organizations, and National Sports Organizations for the Handicapped. Organizations must meet one of three qualifications for membership. The organization must (1) take an active part in the administration of one or more sports or competitions on the Olympic or Pan American Games programs; (2) engage in efforts to promote participation in, or preparation for, amateur athletic competitions, or (3) administer the participation in, or preparation for, professional sports as well as a bona fide program of amateur athletic competition (such as the US Tennis Association). Purely commercial or political organizations are ineligible for membership in the USOC.

Group A (National Governing Bodies)   These organizations are recognized by the USOC as the national governing bodies for sports on the program of the Olympic or Pan American Games and are members of the international federations (IF) recognized by the IOC.

Archery
National Archery Association (NAA)
1750 E Boulder Street
Colorado Springs, CO 80909
(719) 578-4576
IF: Federation Internationale de Tir a l'Arc

Athletics (Track and Field)
The Athletics Congress (TAC)
P.O. Box 120
Indianapolis, IN 46206
(317) 638-9155
IF: International Amateur Athletic Federation (AAF)

Baseball
U.S. Baseball Federation (USBF)
2160 Greenwood Avenue
Trenton, NJ 08609
(609) 586-2381
IF: International Baseball Association (IBA)

Basketball
Amateur Basketball Association of the US (ABAUSA)
1750 E Boulder Street
Colorado Springs, CO 80909
(719) 632-7867
IF: Federation Internationale de Basketball Amateur (FIBA)

Biathlon
U.S. Biathlon Association (USBA)
P.O. Box 5515
Essex Junction, VT 05453
(803) 655-4524
IF: Union Internationale de Pentathlon Moderne et Biathlon (UIPMB)

U.S. Bobsled & Skeleton Association (USBSA)
P.O. Box 828
Lake Placid, NY 12946
(518) 523-1842
IF: Federation Internationale de Bobsleigh et de Tobogganing

Boxing
USA Amateur Boxing Federation (USA/ABF)
1750 E Boulder Street
Colorado Springs, CO 80909
(719) 578-4506
IF: Association Internationale de Boxe Amateur (AIBA)

Canoe/Kayak
American Canoe Association (ACA)
P.O. Box 1190
Newington, VA 22122
(703) 550-7523
IF: Federation Internationale de Canoe (FIC)

National Paddling Committee (NPC)
Pan American Plaza, Suite 470
201 S Capitol Avenue
Indianapolis, IN 46225
(317) 237-5690
(Responsible for Olympic flatwater canoeing and kayaking)

Cycling
U.S. Cycling Federation (USCF)
1750 E Boulder Street
Colorado Springs, CO 80909
(719) 578-4581
IF: Federation Internationale Amateur de Cyclisme (FIAC)

Diving
United States Diving, Inc. (USD)
Pan American Plaza, Suite 430
201 S Capitol Avenue
Indianapolis, IN 46225
(317) 237-5252
IF: Federation Internationale de Natation Amateur (FINA)

Equestrian
American Horse Shows Association (AHSA)
Daily News Building
220 E. 42nd Street, Suite 409
New York, NY 10017-5806
(212) 972-2472
IF: Federation Equestre Internationale (FEI)

U.S. Equestrian Team (USET)
Gladstone, NJ 07934
(201) 234-1251

Fencing
U.S. Fencing Association (USFA)
1750 E Boulder Street
Colorado Springs, CO 80909
(719) 578-4511
IF: Federation Internationale D'Escrime (FIE)

Field Hockey
Field Hockey Association of America (FHAA) (men)
U.S. Field Hockey Association (USFHA) (women)
1750 E Boulder Street
Colorado Springs, CO 80909
(719) 578-4587 (FHAA)
(719) 578-4567 (USFHA)
IF: Federation Internationale de Hockey (FIH)

Figure Skating
U.S. Figure Skating Association (USFSA)
20 First Street
Colorado Springs, CO 80906
(719) 635-5200
International Skating Union (ISU)

Gymnastics (Artistic and Rhythmic)
U.S. Gymnastics Federation (USGF)
Pan American Plaza, Suite 300
201 S Capitol Avenue
Indianapolis, IN 46225
(317) 237-5050
IF: Federation Internationale de Gymnastique (FIG)

Ice Hockey
Amateur Hockey Association of the United States (AHAUS)
2997 Broadmoor Valley Road
Colorado Springs, CO 80906
(719) 576-4990
IF: Internationale Ice Hockey Federation (IIHF)

Judo
United States Judo, Inc. (USJ)
P.O. Box 10013
El Paso, TX 79991
(915) 565-8754
IF: Federation Internationale de Judo (IJE)

Luge
U.S. Luge Association (USLA)
P.O. Box 651
Lake Placid, NY 12946
(518) 523-2071
IF: Federation Internationale de Luge de Course (FIL)

Modern Pentathlon
U.S. Modern Pentathlon Association, Inc. (USMPA)
P.O. Box 8178
San Antonio, TX 78208
(512) 228-0055 or 228-0075
IF: Union Internationale de Pentathlon Moderne et Biathlon (UIPMB)

Roller Skating
U.S. Amateur Confederation of Roller Skating (USAC/RS)
P.O. Box 83067
Lincoln, NE 68501
(402) 483-7551
IF: Federation Internationale de Roller Skating (FIRS)

Rowing
U.S. Rowing Association (USRA)
Pan American Plaza, Suite 400
201 S Capitol Avenue
Indianapolis, IN 46225
(317) 237-5656
IF: Federation Internationale des Societes d'Aviron (FISA)

Shooting
National Rifle Association (NRA)
1600 Rhode Island Avenue, NW
Washington, DC 20036
(202) 828-6000
IF: Union Internationale de Tir (UIT)

Skiing
U.S. Ski Association (USSA)
1750 E Boulder Street
Colorado Springs, CO 80909
(719) 578-4600
IF: Federation Internationale de Ski (FIS)

U.S. Ski Team (USST)
P.O. Box 100
Park City, UT 84060
(801) 649-9090

Soccer (Football)
U.S. Soccer Federation (USSF)
1750 E Boulder Street
Colorado Springs, CO 80909
(719) 578-4678
IF: Federation Internationale de Football Association (FIFA)

Softball
Amateur Softball Association (ASA)
2801 NE 50th Street
Oklahoma City, OK 73111
(405) 424-5266
IF: Federation Internationale de Softball (ISF)

Speed Skating
U.S. International Speedskating Association (USISA)
17060 Patricia Lane
Brookfield, WI 53005
(414) 782-3533
IF: International Skating Union (ISU)

Swimming
U.S. Swimming, Inc. (USS)
1750 E Boulder Street
Colorado Springs, CO 80909
(719) 578-4578
IF: Federation Internationale de Natation Amateur (FINA)

Synchronized Swimming
U.S. Synchronized Swimming, Inc. (USSS)
Pan American Plaza, Suite 510
201 S Capitol Avenue
Indianapolis, IN 46225
(317) 237-5700
IF: Federation Internationale de Natation Amateur (FINA)

Table Tennis
U.S. Table Tennis Association (USTTA)
1750 E Boulder Street
Colorado Springs, CO 80909
(719) 578-4583
IF: International Table Tennis Federation (ITTF)

Tae Kwon Do
U.S. Tae Kwon Do Union (USTU)
1750 E Boulder Street
Colorado Springs, CO 80909
(719) 578-4632
IF: World Tae Kwon Do Federation (WTF)

Team Handball
U.S. Team Handball Federation (USTHF)
1750 E Boulder Street
Colorado Springs, CO 80909
(719) 578-4582
IF: International Handball Federation (IHF)

Tennis
U.S. Tennis Association (USTA)
1212 Avenue of the Americas, 12th Floor
New York, NY 10036
(212) 302-3322
IF: International Tennis Federation (ITF)

Volleyball
U.S. Volleyball Association (USVBA)
1750 E Boulder Street
Colorado Springs, CO 80909
(719) 632-5551, ext. 3312
IF: Federation Internationale de Volleyball (FIVB)

Water Polo
United States Water Polo (USWP)
1750 E Boulder Street
Colorado Springs, CO 80909
(719) 578-4549
IF: Federation Internationale de Natation Amateur (FINA)

Weightlifting
U.S. Weightlifting Federation (USWF)
1750 E Boulder Street
Colorado Springs, CO 80909
(719) 578-4508
IF: International Weightlifting Federation (IWF)

Wrestling
U.S.A. Wrestling
405 W Hall of Fame Avenue
Stillwater, OK 74075
(405) 377-5242
IF: Federation Internationale de Lutte Amateur (FILA)

Yachting
U.S. Yacht Racing Union (USYRU)
P.O. Box 209
Newport, RI 02840
(401) 849-5200
IF: International Yacht Racing Union (IYRU)

Group B (National Multi-Sports Organizations) These organizations directly or indirectly conduct a national program or regular national amateur athletic competition in two or more sports that are included on the programs of the Olympic or Pan American Games.

Amateur Athletic Union (AAU)
3400 W 86th Street
P.O. Box 68207
Indianapolis, IN 46268
(317) 476-2900

American Alliance for Health, Physical Education, Recreation and Dance (AAHPERD)
1900 Association Drive
Reston, VA 22091
(703) 476-3400

Boys Clubs of America
National Olympic Sports Programs Headquarters
10520 Magnolia Blvd
North Hollywood, CA 91601
(818) 506-8033

Catholic Youth Organization (CYO)
1101 First Avenue
New York, NY 10022
(212) 371-1000

Jewish Welfare Board (JWB)
15 E 26th Street
New York, NY 10010
(212) 532-4949

National Association of Intercollegiate Athletics (NAIA)
1221 Baltimore
Kansas City, MO 64105
(816) 842-5050

National Collegiate Athletic Association (NCAA)
P.O. Box 1906
Mission, KS 66201
(913) 384-3220

National Exploring Division, Boy Scouts of America
1325 Walnut Hill Lane
Irving, TX 75038-3096
(214) 580-2423

National Federation of State High School Associations (NFSHSA)
P.O. Box 20626
Kansas City, MO 64195
(816) 464-5400

National Junior College Athletic Association (NJCAA)
P.O. Box 7305
Colorado Springs, CO 80933-7305
(719) 590-9788

US Armed Forces (Air Force, Army, Marine Corps, and Navy)
Hoffman Building 1, Room 1416
2461 Eisenhower Avenue
Alexandria, VA 22331
(202) 325-8871

Young Men's Christian Association of the USA (YMCA)
101 N Wacker Drive
Chicago, IL 60606
(312) 977-0031

Group C (Affiliated Sports Organizations) These organizations are ineligible to be Group A members, but function as national governing bodies in amateur sports that are not on the current program of the Olympic or Pan American Games. (The badminton and bowling organizations will become Group A members in the 1989–1992 quadrennium.)

Badminton
US Badminton Association (USBA)
501 W 6th Street
Papillion, NE 68046
(402) 592-7309
IF: International Badminton Federation (IBF)

Bowling
American Bowling Congress (ABC) (men)
Women's International Bowling Congress (WIBC)
5301 S 76th Street
Greendale, WI 53129
(414) 421-6400 (ABC)
(414) 421-9000 (WIBC)
IF: Federation Internationale des Quilleurs (FIQ)

Curling
US Curling Association (USCA)
1100 Center Pont Drive
Box 972
Stevens Point, WI 54481
(715) 344-1199
IF: International Curling Federation (ICF)

Karate
The USA Karate Federation (USAKF)
1300 Kenmore Blvd
Akron, OH 44314
(216) 753-3114
IF: World Union of Karatedo Organizations (WUKO)

Racquetball
American Amateur Racquetball Association (AARA)
815 N Weber, Suite 101
Colorado Springs, CO 80903
(719) 635-5396
IF: International Amateur Racquetball Federation (IARF)

Sports Acrobatics
United States Sports Acrobatics Federation
5538 S Marine Drive
Tempoe, AZ 85283
(602) 249-4002
IF: International Federation of Sports Acrobatics (IFSA)

Water Skiing
American Water Ski Association (AWSA)
P.O. Box 191
Winter Haven, FL 33882
(813) 324-4341
IF: Union Mondiale de Ski Nauique (UMSN)

Group D (State Olympic Organizations) These Olympic organizations for each state and the District of Columbia are recognized by the USOC and bring together interested individuals, organizations, and corporations to further the purposes and goals of the Olympic movement in the United States. These organizations conduct and coordinate USOC fund-raising activities and enhance the image of the USOC by establishing broad, comprehensive communications programs so that the general public can more readily identify with the Olympic movement.

Group E (National Sports Organizations for the Handicapped) These amateur organizations are ineligible for another class of membership in the USOC, but conduct a national program or regular national athletic competition in two or more sports on the program of the Olympic or Pan American Games.

American Athletic Association of the Deaf (AAAD)
1134 Davenport Drive
Burton, MI 48529
(313) 239-3962

United States Amputee Athletic Association (USSAAA)
Belle Forest Circle, Suite 149-A
Nashville, TN 37221
(615) 662-2323

US Association for Blind Athletes (USABA)
UAF/USC Benson Building
Columbia, SC 29208
(803) 777-4465

Untied States Cerebral Palsy Athletic Association (USCPAA)
34518 S Warren Road, Suite 264
Westland, MI 48185
(313) 425-8961

National Handicapped Sports and Recreation Association
        (NHSRA)
Capitol Hill Station
P.O. Box 18664
Denver, CO 18664
(303) 232-4575

National Wheelchair Athletic Association (NWAA)
3617 Betty Drive, Suite S
Colorado Springs, CO 80917
(719) 597-8330

Special Olympics, Inc.
1350 New York Avenue, NW
Suite 500
Washington, DC 20005 (202) 628-3630

Consensus Statements:
Pediatric Sport Psychology and Sport Organization

1. Definitive sports' structures have evolved over the past 100 years. Many of us question whether these organizations are meeting the needs of children. In some instances sports have become too competitive and children are experiencing burnout. Sport psychologists have become involved with the pediatric athlete, and some promising changes have been made to rectify these problems.

2. It is important for all persons involved in youth sports to have some knowledge of youth-sport organizations and of the role of pediatric psychology in the management of the pediatric athlete. This knowledge is also important in the training of the youth-sport coach and of the sports medicine physician.

3. While the manner in which role models develop is poorly understood, it is clear that children often emulate elite athletes. These role models are critical to how a young person approaches participation in sports. A role model conveys to the individual the importance of exercise, fitness, and sports as leisure-time activities. One's approach to life in general is also influenced by these role models.

Section Five

Musculoskeletal Injury

Chapter 16

Epidemiology of Sports Injuries in the Pediatric Athlete

James G. Garrick, MD

The goal of sports medicine is to prevent injuries, or, failing that, to provide prompt, appropriate medical care for the injured. Although most individuals would agree this objective is desirable, meaningful cooperative efforts to achieve this goal have been infrequent, sometimes haphazard, and often unscientific.

Preventing sports injuries and providing appropriate medical care for athletes require medically and scientifically reliable information about both the injury and the circumstances surrounding its occurrence. However, obtaining such information has proved difficult in the sports arena where emotions run high, traditions are sacrosanct, and medical practice is often viewed with some suspicion. In addition, sport or "playing games" is often viewed as a frivolous activity. Nonetheless, no other activity consumes as much time or involves as many people as sports, and still society is medically ignorant of prevention and treatment of sports injuries.

There is little medical research on sports injuries, and children's athletic injuries are the subject of a disproportionate amount of this research. However, this research is heavily influenced by the nature of the injury and the sport involved. For example, the medical and legal attention paid to permanent cervical spinal cord injuries sustained in high-school football has caused some to question the wisdom of allowing children to play this sport even though hundreds more such injuries are sustained by diving into shallow water; indeed, they occurred four times more often in men's gymnastics than in high-school football.[1]

Knowledge about the medical aspects of sports is idiosyncratic, leaning heavily toward highly visible sports (football), rapidly emerging sports (soccer), catastrophic injuries (blindness and cervical spine injuries), and injuries that involve economic interests (the cost effectiveness of knee braces).

Epidemiologic Issues

The epidemiologic study of youth sports encompasses traditional issues such as appropriate study design, avoiding bias, identifying the population at risk, and developing an appropriate definition of injury. On the surface, youth sports should provide fertile ground for epidemiologic investigation. These activities are usually organized somewhat formally, participation is documented, and adult—even professional—supervision is usually present. Nevertheless, it is difficult to obtain the quality and quantity of information necessary for a successful epidemiologic study.

Injury Definition and Recognition

The major difficulty is defining the injury in a manner that is both medically meaningful and functionally realistic. In youth sports, methods of identifying and recording injuries depend almost entirely on the abilities and experience of those supervising the activity.

The coach is the ideal person to identify and record the presence of injuries. The coach is not only in a position to observe the occurrence of the injury, but also, as the adult authority present, to disseminate medical advice. However, because the coach is also responsible for the conduct and performance of the team, injuries that are not obvious or disabling may be underestimated and underreported. Goldberg and associates,[2] for example, found that only slightly more than half (55.2%) of the time-loss injuries (injuries causing the athlete to miss practice or competition) reported by athletes and their parents were also reported by coaches and administrators in a Pop Warner football league.

Team insurance claims are often used to define and report injuries. Injuries requiring medical treatment and reported under insurance claims are "significant." However, this means that formal medical care was sought and given and the claim filed with the insurance company. Yet "team insurance" is often treated as secondary coverage, used only if the child does not have a primary carrier or if the costs are beyond those covered by personal insurance. These factors may explain why Roser and Clawson[3] reported that only 2.3% of the 9- to 15-year-old participants in the Seattle Junior Football Program were injured (data obtained from coaching reports and insurance claims), whereas Goldberg and associates[2] reported that 15.4% were injured (data obtained from interviews with the athletes and their parents).

These two studies illustrate some of the difficulties in identifying and recording the injuries sustained by children during athletic activities. Although both investigations involved football players, the same problems undoubtedly exist in other athletic activities, such as soccer, baseball, swimming, gymnastics, and even dance. Studies of such activities should include direct contact with the athletes and their parents.

Conventional wisdom suggests that injury reporting is more reliable in institution-sponsored sports. Although some middle and junior high schools offer interscholastic athletic activities, most of these programs exist at the high-school level. There, coaches are more likely to have formal training, lines of authority and responsibility exist, the contact between coach and athlete is more frequent, and the fear of legal reprisals is more compelling. Additionally, high-school athletic programs

Table 1. Comparative Injury Rate[4]

Sport	Injuries per 100 Participants	
	No.	No. Resulting in > 5 Days Lost
Baseball (boys)	19	4.5
Basketball (boys)	31	7.4
Football (boys)	81	25.1
Track and field (boys)	33	12.5
Track and field (girls)	35	17.5
Wrestling (boys)	75	26.3

are more likely to include the services of an athletic trainer—the best person to recognize and report injuries.

With the presence of more medically sophisticated personnel, such as athletic trainers, record-keeping improves and it becomes possible to define injury more precisely and to establish comparative injury rates among sports (Table 1). Garrick and Requa[4] used athletic trainers at four high schools to identify, classify, and record athletic injuries. During the two-year investigation, there were 1,197 injuries in 3,049 participants. Injuries were defined as medical conditions arising from sports participation that caused the athlete to discontinue activity in a practice or competitive event or miss a subsequent practice or event. Although these data have limited value in preventing specific injuries, it can be used to help determine necessary medical coverage for sports or events.

Injuries by Sport

Comparing a football game to a tennis match shows the quantitative and the qualitative differences in injury potential between athletic activities. Less striking, but perhaps equally important from an epidemiologic standpoint, is the functional disability associated with the same injury in different sports. For example, a sprained finger might be little more than a nuisance to the football player yet be totally disabling for a tennis player. It is therefore important to view injuries in the context of the sport involved.

One method of examining the importance of an injury is the time lost from athletic participation. Although physicians view injuries in terms of pathology and location, athletes, parents, and coaches take a more pragmatic approach. The fact that the athlete asks "When can I play again?" rather than "How bad is the injury?" is testimony to this pragmatism.

In the Garrick and Requa study, one of the "severity indices" was a measure of time lost to athletic participation. For example, the overall injury rate among football players was 81 injuries per 100 participants per season. Only 31% of these injuries resulted in time-loss exceeding five days (25 injuries per 100 participants). The percentages of injury resulting in more than five days of time lost varied widely among sports, from a low of none in badminton and boys gymnastics to a high of 57% in boys' cross-country track and girls' swimming. Overall, 26.6% of the injuries resulted in more than five days of time lost. Table 1 shows the total number of injuries and the number of injuries that resulted in more than five days of time lost for the most popular sports (those with more than 200 participants during the course of the investigation).

Although in general the ranking of sports by degree of safety (or danger) does not change greatly when considering only injuries resulting in more than five days lost, there are a few instances in which the ranking changed appreciably. Boys' cross-country track and girls' track-and-field, for example, become two of the most hazardous sports, ranking third and fourth after football and wrestling.

Injury by Age

Controversy surrounds the issue of age and participation in organized sports. One cannot help but question the propriety of sending a 9-year-old out to play football after studying injury statistics drawn from the professional and college levels. Yet, it appears that the safety implications in football—as well as in soccer and in baseball—are strikingly different for children and adults.

It is difficult to compare injury rates for various organizational levels of sports participation, primarily because of reporting difficulties. Nonetheless, when roughly similar definitions of injury exist, there appear to be substantial differences between the injury rates in sports for children and young teenagers and those in interscholastic sports at the high-school level.

In the Pop Warner football program studied by Goldberg and associates,[2] the rates of "significant" injuries (more than seven days lost) were 2.8 per 100 participants for 9- to 12-year-olds, 3.7 per 100 for 10- to 13-year-olds, and 10.1 per 100 for 11- to 14-year-olds, for an overall average of 5.7 per 100. Yet the rate of "significant" injuries (more than five days lost) derived from the Seattle High School study[3] was more than four times higher (25 per 100 participants).

Both Goldberg and associates[2] and Robey and associates[5] examined the apparent influence of age within a specific organizational framework in which definitions of injury and data collection were, presumably, consistent (Figs. 1 and 2). Sullivan and associates[6] examined injury statistics from a youth soccer program in Oklahoma, using a definition of injury similar to that employed by Goldberg and associates. From this information, they calculated injury rates for players of various ages (Fig. 3).

A consistent pattern emerged showing that injury rates increased with age. The fact that the oldest group in each study had somewhat lower injury rates may have been related to the relatively small number of participants.

One explanation for the higher injury rates in high-school football players may be the increased time at risk. At the high-school level, games

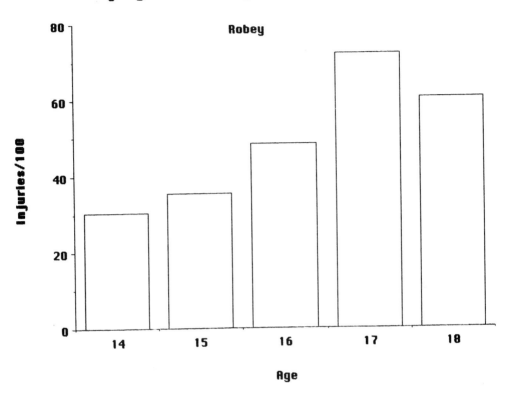

Fig. 1 *Injury rates in high-school football.*[5]

last longer and practices are more frequent, giving the player more opportunities to be injured. Additionally, with medical care more readily available at the high-school level, injuries are more likely to be reported.

It seems unlikely that any physiologic or anatomic factor associated with increasing age is responsible for an enhanced likelihood of injury. Indeed, conventional wisdom suggests the contrary, since the participants in the younger groups are skeletally immature.

Factors that may explain this finding include the larger size, increased speed, and greater skill of the older players. In a contact sport such as football, both size and speed increase the forces involved in collisions, perhaps making these collisions more hazardous. Although collisions do occur in soccer, noncontact injuries would seem to be more likely, but the same pattern of increasing injury rates associated with increasing age occurs in both sports.

As players increase in age and expertise, they must go through a more rigorous selection process for team membership. One of the major

Injury Rates in Youth Football

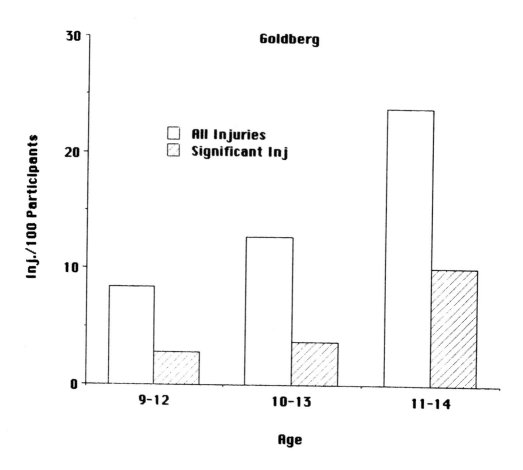

Fig. 2 *Injury rates in youth football.*[2]

goals of most youth sport programs should be to provide an opportunity for everyone to play regardless of ability; interscholastic high-school programs, however, are much more oriented toward team success and winning. Thus, team members are selected on the basis of athletic skills that often include characteristics associated with increased risk of injury. For example, the football coach who seeks players who are "punishing tacklers" probably inadvertently encourages higher injury rates. Although greater athletic proficiency may convey some safety benefits in soccer and football, as it does in skiing, these benefits may not help the opponent. For example, increased expertise might well make slide tackling in soccer or tackling in football safer for the tackler but more haz-

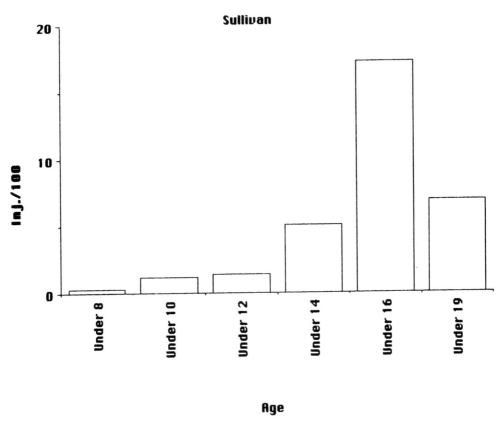

Fig. 3 *Injury rates in youth soccer.*[6]

ardous for the player being tackled. Requa and Garrick[7] noted a similar situation in high-school wrestlers, who were more likely to sustain injuries when they were "down."

Injuries by Type

If the ultimate goal is injury prevention, medically accurate diagnoses are essential. A medically accurate description of an injury provides critical information regarding its cause. For example, to study the effectiveness of prophylactic knee braces it is essential that knee sprains be identified. Similarly, any protective influence offered by pregame stretching will be missed if strains are not specifically recorded. All too often injuries are categorized by anatomic region alone; thus, the "leg injury" of a soccer player might be the result of inadequate stretching or warm-up (strain) or of not wearing shin guards (contusion).

Unfortunately pathologic precision is commonly lacking in injury studies, especially those reported by nonmedical investigators. The relatively common practice of combining sprains and strains or fractures and dislocations makes such information almost meaningless in an epidemiologic sense.

Most injury-reporting systems are most sensitive to injuries that are immediately obvious and disabling. Thus, fractures, lacerations, and severe sprains and strains readily find their way into most reporting schemes. Conditions that result in delayed disability, such as moderate sprains and strains, some subluxations, and deep contusions, become "injuries" by virtue of subsequent missed practices or games and are more likely to escape detection.

Many nonmedical observers consider so-called minor injuries as unimportant because they are not disabling or do not result in any appreciable lost time. Although this may be true from the coach's standpoint, the epidemiologist views these injuries in a different light. With the possible exception of fractures, most sports injuries encompass a broad range of severity levels. The epidemiologic importance of the injury is related to what structures are injured rather than to how badly they are injured; thus, a "minor" injury counts as much as a major one. Because minor injuries occur more frequently than major ones, a reporting system that ignores these problems reduces the numbers in the data pool, decreasing its usefulness.

The identification of injuries without regard to their severity is also important in assessing programs intended to enhance safety. "Injury prevention" in many cases is actually injury attenuation. It is unlikely, for example, that the use of prophylactic knee braces in football or of ankle taping in basketball will prevent knee or ankle sprains, because these devices do not alter the circumstance causing the injury. Rather, such measures are meant to reduce the magnitude of the forces applied to the ligament, thus converting a grade III sprain to a grade II sprain and a grade II sprain to a grade I sprain. Because the more severe (grade III) injuries are so few, documenting the efficacy of such practices may be impossible without including the larger numbers of less severe injuries.

Categorizing injuries by their pathologies can suggest potential causes of sports injury and help evaluate methods of injury prevention. It can also provide valuable insight on the actual conduct and validity of epidemiologic study. Fractures, because of their obvious nature, are perhaps the most reliably reported common sport injury. Thus, the number of fractures in the total injury pool provides some insight into the frequency of reporting for other injuries. A study by Garrick and Requa[4] of 19 high-school sports reported 5.3% of the injuries as fractures (5.8% in football); Sullivan and associates[6] (youth soccer) found 5.9% fractures; McMaster and Walter[8] (adult soccer) reported 2.9% fractures; Goldberg and associates[2] (youth football) reported 14.9% fractures, and

Roser and Clawson[3] (youth football) found 35% fractures. Viewed singly, the report by Roser and Clawson suggests that youth football in Seattle in the 1960s was beset with some appreciable problems. Comparing the methodology of the studies, however, shows that the rate of occurrence of fractures in the Roser and Clawson study was 0.82 per 100 participants,[3] whereas that in the study by Goldberg and associates was 2.29 per 100.[2] So, instead of indicating an inordinately high incidence of severe injuries (fractures), the "35% fractures" statistic suggests that other injuries were underreported.

Finally, it is nearly impossible to characterize injury patterns within a specific sport without precise pathologic classifications. In the Garrick and Requa[4] study, the injury rates for boys' basketball and boys' cross-country track were almost identical (31 and 29 per 100 participants, respectively). Even an unsophisticated observer would realize that the demands of and the injuries in these activities are entirely different. Basketball involves quick bursts of activity, the ability to sprint, jump, and turn sharply, and frequent contact and collisions. Cross-country running, on the other hand, requires aerobic endurance and long hours of repetitious practice of a single act—running. Playing basketball results in a variety of injuries (sprains, strains, and contusions), most of which are acute. Cross-country running is more likely to produce injuries with a gradual onset (overuse injuries).

To the epidemiologist, overuse injuries present perhaps the greatest challenge as well as the greatest opportunity to change behavior. Whereas acute injuries are frequently random (the player is in the wrong place at the wrong time), overuse injuries are usually the result of "training errors" (doing the wrong thing). Thus, the circumstances surrounding overuse injuries lend themselves more readily to change and, ultimately, prevention.

The major problem associated with studying overuse injuries is identifying them. At the onset, overuse injuries are only subtly disabling, unlike the immediate fall to the ground that accompanies an ankle sprain. Signs and symptoms are often vague and discovering them requires a great deal of sophistication, often well beyond the capabilities of the nonmedical observer.

Thus, a lack of medical precision in recognizing and diagnosing overuse injuries results in underestimating the hazards associated with some athletic activities. More importantly, the coach and athlete are unable to prevent injuries that should be among the most preventable. Such conditions as spondylolysis in female gymnasts and osteochondritis dissecans of the Little Leaguer's elbow are examples of these injuries. Overuse injuries must not be dismissed as "nuisance problems" of little medical consequence.

Summary

Epidemiology plays a crucial role in every aspect of sports medicine. Those who teach sports must know what injuries are associated with a particular sport. Knowing what injuries are likely to occur makes it easier to prepare medical coverage for an athletic event. Precise medical information is needed to evaluate the efficacy of programs intended to prevent injuries and to compare treatment regimens. Finally, unless sports medicine takes the sound, scientific approach used in other, more traditional medical areas, the care of athletes will continue to be regarded with less urgency than it deserves. Preserving the health of those fit enough to play games merits the same scientific commitment as does attempting to cure the ill.

References

1. Torg JS: *Athletic Injuries to the Head, Neck and Face*. Philadelphia, Lea and Febiger, 1982, pp 18-20.
2. Goldberg B, Rosenthal PP, Nicholas JA: Injuries in youth football. *Phys Sportsmed* 1984;12:122-132.
3. Roser LA, Clawson DK: Football injuries in the very young athlete. *Clin Orthop* 1970;69:219-223.
4. Garrick JG, Requa RK: Injuries in high school sports. *Pediatrics* 1978;61:465-469.
5. Robey JM, Blyth CS, Mueller FO: Athletic injuries. Application of epidemiologic methods. *JAMA* 1971;217:184-189.
6. Sullivan JA, Gross RH, Grana WA, et al: Evaluation of injuries in youth soccer. *Am J Sports Med* 1980;8:325-327.
7. Requa R, Garrick JG: Injuries in interscholastic wrestling. *Phys Sportsmed* 1981;9:44-51.
8. McMaster WC, Walter M: Injuries in soccer. *Am J Sports Med* 1978;6:354-357.

Chapter 17

Injuries to the Head, Neck, and Spine

William A. Herndon, MD

Severe head or neck injury is a catastrophe to the patient, the patient's family, and society. The incidence of major head or spinal cord injury in children under 15 years old is low, but increases significantly in those 15 to 18 years old.[1] Severe head injury is most common in motor-vehicle accidents and falls.[2-4] The incidence of head injury in contact sports, although significant, has decreased with changes in equipment so that sports-related spinal cord injuries now receive much more attention. Most spinal cord injuries occur as a result of motor-vehicle accidents (38%), falls or jumps (16%), and gunshot wounds (13%).[5] Sports-related spinal cord injuries are less common. Only diving (9%) is responsible for a significant number of injuries. American football and trampoline injuries each account for approximately 1% of all spinal cord injuries, while ice hockey, rugby, and gymnastic activities each account for less than 1%. Although these percentages may seem small, the relative risks to participants in football, gymnastics, rugby, and ice hockey are unknown because the number of people exposed to possible injury is difficult to determine.

Most sports-related spinal injuries involve the cervical spine.[6] Motor-vehicle accidents and falls produce roughly equal numbers of paraplegics and quadriplegics, whereas sports injuries more often produce quadriplegic patients. Ninety-eight percent of diving injuries and 80% of other sports injuries to the cervical spine result in quadriplegia.

Spinal cord injuries recently became a reportable condition in the state of Oklahoma. From October 1987 through August 1988, 127 traumatic spinal cord injuries were reported. Motor-vehicle accidents accounted for more than half of these injuries. Eleven people had sports-related spinal cord injuries. Eight of the 127 patients (6%) were injured in diving accidents. There was one football injury, one boxing injury, and one rodeo injury. No injuries occurred in children under 16 years old.

According to available statistics, 5% of diving injuries occur in children under 15 years old and 83% occur in people 15 to 29 years old.[6]

These percentages are similar to those for other sports and to those for motor-vehicle accidents and penetrating wounds.

Does the large difference in injuries between age groups imply a difference in the number of patients at risk or a difference in the susceptibility of younger patients to brain or spinal cord injury? Kalsbeek and associates[3] indicated that brain injury was less common in younger individuals. The incidence of significant injury in children under 15 years old is 230 per 100,000; the incidence in those 15 to 24 years old is 349 per 100,000. However, this probably represents a difference in the number of patients at risk rather than a difference in susceptibility to injury.

A study of 75 patients with spinal cord injuries from birth through 18 years of age at Children's Hospital of Oklahoma[5] demonstrated the following: (1) children usually had spinal cord injury without evidence of osseous fracture (birth through 15 years); (2) children and adolescents (11 to 18 years old) tended to have fractures that were apparent on radiographs; (3) all the children had been involved in motor-vehicle accidents; and (4) 13% of the adolescent injuries were caused by diving and 1% of the injuries were caused by trampoline use. During the same period, femoral fractures treated at the same institution were evenly spread over all age groups. Because both femoral fractures and spinal cord injuries are the result of significant trauma, it can be concluded that the immature spine may be more resistant to spinal cord injury.

Statistics from the National Football Head and Neck Injury Registry[7] also indicate that the incidence of sports-related spinal cord injuries increases with age. In 1984 cervical spine injuries occurred in 3.9 per 100,000 participants in high school and 6.73 per 100,000 in college. However, factors such as the number of players at risk, experience, body weight, and velocity of performance all play a role in the differing incidences of injury in different age groups. Nevertheless, it is likely that younger spines are less susceptible to injury.

Football

American football is the most common collision sport for children and adolescents. It has the highest incidence of injuries of all sports in elementary, junior, and senior high school.[1]

Head and spinal injuries in athletes have been best studied in football players. These studies prove the value of epidemiology in sports. Data on the frequency and mechanism of injury have led to improvements in equipment and rule changes that dramatically improved safety. Although severe injuries are rare, the evidence[8] suggests that as many as one-third of participants in organized football at the college level have radiographic evidence of cervical spine injury.

In 1975 the National Football Head and Neck Injury Registry was established to gather accurate statistics. The initial study[9] retrospectively looked at intracranial hemorrhage, intracranial injuries resulting in death, cervical fractures, subluxations and dislocations, and cervical spine fracture-dislocations with permanent quadriplegia. This study found a decrease in intracranial lesions and death and an increase in quadriplegia when data from 1971 to 1975 were compared with data from 1959 to 1963. The decrease in head injuries was attributed to new developments in helmet design. It had been postulated that helmets contribute to cervical injury because (1) the face mask forces the neck into severe hyperflexion or (2) the posterior rim of the helmet acts as a "guillotine" when the neck is forced into hyperextension. After some study,[9-11] neither theory has been substantiated.

Bauze and Ardran[12] demonstrated that axial compression applied to the flexed spine produces cervical dislocations. More recent evidence[7,13,14] concerning the pathomechanics of cervical spine injuries in football has shown that axial loading of the slightly flexed neck is responsible for most of these injuries. Better protective headgear allows players to use their heads for blocking, tackling, and butting opponents. Defensive backs, linebackers, and specialty team members who use their heads to ram opponents while tackling them are at the greatest risk.

These findings resulted in rule changes adopted by the National Collegic Athletic Association and the National Federation of State High School Athletic Associations in 1976. The new rules state (1) that no player should intentionally strike a runner with the crown or the top of the helmet, (2) that spearing is a deliberate use of the helmet in an attempt to punish an opponent, and (3) that no player should deliberately use his helmet to butt or ram an opponent.

A prospective study[7] conducted by the National Football Head and Neck Injury Registry at the University of Pennsylvania Sports Medicine Center showed interesting trends. An increase in head injuries was actually documented from 1976 through 1984, but the death rate from intracranial injury remained stable. This was attributed to the advent of computed tomographic scanning, a technique that more accurately diagnoses head injuries. Cervical spine injuries gradually declined from 6.5 per 100,000 high-school players and 29.3 per 100,000 college players to 3.9 per 100,000 and 6.7 per 100,000, respectively. The incidence of permanent quadriplegia was significantly lower in 1984. In 1975, 2.2 per 100,000 high-school players and 8.4 per 100,000 college players became quadriplegic. In 1984 the comparable figures were 0.43 per 100,000 and 0 per 100,000, respectively. The number of injuries causing quadriplegia was 34 in 1976, 18 in 1977, and five in 1984. There is no question that organized football is hazardous, but better equipment and rule changes have certainly made it safer. However, although changes in helmet design have greatly decreased the incidence of serious head injuries, only changes in tackling techniques can lessen the incidence of spinal injuries.

Football players have also been shown to be at risk for less severe lumbar spine injuries.[15] Ferguson and associates,[16] McCarroll and associates,[17] and Cantu[18] demonstrated that interior linemen are at risk for low back sprains and even pars interarticularis injury. Hyperextension of the lumbar spine during blocking has been implicated as the etiologic factor. It is likely that these changes develop early in the player's career.

Diving

Although spinal cord injuries from football have received the most attention in the literature, spinal cord injuries from diving are many times more common. Burke[19] reported on 52 cases of cervical spine injury caused by diving accidents in Australia. Forty-eight of the patients were injured when their heads struck the bottom while they were diving into shallow water. The majority of injuries were described as "burst" fractures.

Kewalramani and associates[20] described 23 diving injuries in patients ranging in age from 15 to 47 years. This series represented 18% of the spinal injuries admitted to their hospital over a three-year period. Neurologic deficit was seen in 21 of the patients. One patient had a head injury in addition to the spinal injury and died as a result. There were 29 fractures in the 23 patients: 15 wedge fractures, seven burst fractures, and seven tear-drop fractures. The authors concluded that flexion was the main force involved in most of the injuries. Only four patients had objective evidence of hitting the bottom and some (less than half) denied hitting the bottom at all. The authors concluded that "we must look for possible force mechanisms resulting from the resistance of the water partially counteracting the momentum of the falling body."

Tator and associates[21] described 38 patients with spinal cord injuries caused by diving accidents. These cases constituted 11% of their entire series of spinal cord injuries. Most injuries occurred in summer. The most common bony injury was posterior fracture dislocation (37%). Anterior fracture dislocations accounted for 24% of the injuries, compression fractures 18%, burst fractures 3%, no bony injury 5%, anterior dislocation 5%, and body fractures 1%. They concluded that the injury occurred "when the top of the head struck the bottom of the lake or pool and not when the head struck the water."

Shields and associates,[22] in discussing spinal cord injuries in athletes, found that 118 of 152 patients with cervical cord injuries were injured while participating in water sports. Diving accidents were the most common. The authors did not detail the mechanism of injury but stated that most of the injuries occurred because the patient dived into shallow water or struck a submerged object after misjudging the depth, which in this series averaged 5 feet.

Albrand and Walter[23] recognized that experienced divers protect their heads with the arms but inexperienced divers often do not. In a retrospective study, 13 of 25 patients responded to a questionnaire. Each had an associated head injury and ten of the 13 lost consciousness at the time of injury. Interestingly, only four of the 13 remembered striking the bottom. The results of this clinical study prompted the authors to film two expert divers to determine velocity rates as they moved through the water. They noted that the velocity did not dissipate until the diver reached a depth of 10 to 12 feet.

The Centers for Disease Control noted an increase in diving-related spinal cord injuries concomitant with the summer drought of 1988.[24]

They emphasized the hazards of diving into natural bodies of water without objective evidence of the depth and advocated public education, posted warnings, and better state surveillance to identify problem areas.

Diving injuries are by far the leading cause of serious spinal injuries in sports. Although there is still some controversy, it appears that the majority of these injuries occur when the head strikes the bottom or an object. This leads to a combination of flexion and axial compression forces that may produce a number of different bony injury patterns. Resulting neurologic injury is common.

Trampoline

Most cervical spine injuries in gymnastics have been sustained on the trampoline and minitrampoline. Numerous reports have focused on the danger of this apparatus. Zimmerman[25] initially described two patients and Ellis and associates[26] described two patients with head injuries and three with spinal cord injuries from the trampoline. Torg and Das[14,27] summarized reports in the European literature[28-31] that described serious neurologic injuries, even in expert gymnasts. In the 1970s more cases were reported in American literature.[32-34] After these reports and the series described by Clarke,[35] the Committee on Accident and Poison Prevention of the American Academy of Pediatrics[36] issued a policy statement that recommended that "trampolines be banned from use as part of the physical education programs in grammar schools, high schools and colleges and also be abolished as a competitive sport."

A National Catastrophic Injury Registry,[37] established in 1978 at the University of Illinois, identified a decrease in the rate of injury in gymnastics and trampoline use after 1978. This was thought to be the result of removing trampolines from schools. Ironically, the American Academy of Pediatrics[38] later changed its policy somewhat. The new policy states:

The trampoline is a potentially dangerous apparatus, and its use demands the following precautions:

1. The trampoline should not be a part of routine physical education classes.

2. The trampoline has no place in competitive sports.

3. The trampoline should never be used in home or recreational settings.

4. Highly trained personnel who have been instructed in all aspects of trampoline safety must be present when the apparatus is used.

5. Maneuvers, especially the somersaults, that have a high potential for serious injury should be attempted only by those qualified to become skilled performers.

6. The trampoline must be secured when not in use, and it must be well maintained.

7. Only schools or sports activities complying with the foregoing recommendations should have trampolines.

Torg and Das[27] take a stronger stand. Although no data exist to determine the risk of injury on the basis of the number of individuals exposed, they state that at least 114 cases of quadriplegia have been described as being secondary to trampoline or minitrampoline use. In addition, some participants experienced an unexplained "blackout" just before the injury.[28] Furthermore, as documented in the Christensen and Clarke[37] series, many cases involved skilled trampolinists attempting to perform a forward or backward somersault. Torg and Das believe that in many cases injuries are not preventable and even expert supervision and coaching, as well as better equipment, will not prevent catastrophic spinal cord injuries. They conclude, "Both the trampoline and mini-trampoline are dangerous devices when used in the best of circumstances, and their use has no place in recreational, educational, or competitive gymnastics."

Gymnastics

Although most gymnastics-related injuries occur on the trampoline, head and neck injuries have been seen after falls from other types of apparatus.[35] The 1982 world champion of women's gymnastics is now a quadriplegic.[39]

Less severe injuries to the spine have received the most attention, however.[15,40] Jackson and associates[40] reported that lumbar spine injuries were very common in female gymnasts. They found an incidence of spondylolysis of 11%, compared with 2.3% in the general population. The increased incidence of pars interarticularis defects was attributed to fatigue-loading of the posterior elements of the low lumbar spine. Both Garrick and Requa[41] and Jackson and associates[40] believe that the hyperlordotic posture and hyperextension required in many gymnastic routines lead to a high incidence of back strains and sprains. Maximal strengthening of the abdominal and spinal extensor musculature is the recommended preventive measure.

Ice Hockey

Attention was first called to neurologic injury in hockey in 1968 with a report on severe brain injuries[42] attributed to inadequate helmets. Feriencik,[43] in a review of ice hockey injuries, did not call attention to spinal cord injuries. Tator and associates[44,45] more recently reported 42 spinal injuries in Canada between 1976 and 1983. Twenty-eight of these players had spinal cord injuries; 17 had complete injuries. Between 1974 and 1983 six patients were treated, a marked contrast to the period 1948–1973 when no injuries were reported. Most injuries occurred during organized hockey play and involved players at all levels. A direct blow to the head was responsible for every injury. The head struck the boards in 25 instances, other players in six, a combination of the boards and other players in four, and the goal post in one. The remaining six players did not know what object was struck. The figures supported the claim by Tator and associates that the incidence of spinal cord injury was increasing in the sport.

The victims were in their teens or early 20s and played in organized leagues. The mechanism of injury was axial compression with slight flexion. The authors stated that, on a per capita basis, hockey in Canada was responsible for three times as much quadriplegia as American football. They offered several recommendations, including better enforcement of the rules, especially those against boarding and crosschecking; consideration of new rules against pushing or checking from behind; cervical muscle-strengthening exercises; player education to avoid spearing and impact, especially against the boards with the neck flexed; research on helmet design; and further research on the biomechanics of the injuries.

Gerberich and associates[46] found that 22% of all injuries sustained in high-school ice hockey were of the head and neck. Sim and associates[47] attributed the increase in neck and spinal cord injuries to the development of a better helmet in response to the previous high incidence of head and facial injuries. Biomechanical studies[48,49] do not support the view that a heavy helmet places more stress on the cervical spine.

It appears that cervical spine problems in hockey players have paralleled those in football players. With the development of better headgear to protect against brain injury,[50] the incidence of spinal injuries has increased. The mechanism of injury is much the same—a severe axial compression force applied to the slightly flexed head.

Rugby

Rugby is the primary collision sport outside the United States. Interestingly enough, despite the lack of protective equipment and the speed of the game, severe head injuries are rare.[1] In 1981, two separate studies detailed spinal injuries sustained in rugby football. Scher[51] described the case of a player injured while tackling. The mechanism of injury was a blow to the head that caused axial compression with the neck in a slightly flexed position. The author recommended better neck muscle conditioning as a preventive measure.

In a separate study from New Zealand,[52] 54 cases of cervical spine injury were identified from 1973 through 1978. There were five fatalities, 11 permanent injuries, nine cases of temporary quadriplegia, and 29 minor or moderate injuries. One-third of the injuries occurred during training or social games. In 1975, 13 cases were reported, compared with 29 cases from diving injuries and 25 cases from other sports. Formation of the scrum, collapse of the scrum, and loose mauls were all sources of danger. Forwards had twice as many injuries as backs, possibly because of their participation in scrums. Injuries outside the scrum were equally common in forwards and backs. The authors concluded that player education, better coaching, and rule changes might reduce the risk of injury. They also concluded that the incidence of serious injury in rugby did not seem to be increasing.

More recent studies have continued to demonstrate the danger. Taylor and Coolican[53] demonstrated that significant injuries still occur. Scrum engagement, and not scrum collapse, seemed to be the most dangerous. Davidson[54] studied school-age participants and concluded that injuries were not increasing and that rugby was safe for that age group. The above studies concluded that injuries increased with age and experience and that an Australian national registry should be established to delineate the risks of the sport better. Other sound suggestions came from a study conducted in Ireland.[55] It recommended "that teams be matched for weight and skill rather than by age alone; and that dangerous play, such as 'crash' or 'spear' tackling or collapsing the scrum, must be swiftly punished." As in American football, rule changes aimed at curbing dangerous and aggressive play should decrease the risk of serious neural injury.

Wrestling

Wrestling ranks second (behind football) in the incidence of injuries in organized sports. Despite that, there is a low rate of brain and spinal cord injury.[1] In 1951 Gonzales[56] reported that one of two deaths from wrestling resulted from complications of a spinal injury. Leidholt,[57] in 1973, found that 11 of 31 spinal injuries in sports exclusive of football were caused by wrestling. None, however, produced significant neurologic deficit. Wu and Lewis[58] recently described three serious spinal cord injuries sustained in wrestling accidents. One injury was caused by a full nelson hold and the other two injuries occurred when the participants landed on their heads after being thrown. Cervical spine and head injuries appear to be rare in wrestling but occasional severe injuries can and do occur.

Boxing

There is little doubt that boxers are at high risk for serious injury, particularly intracranial hemorrhage.[59] Despite this, severe intracranial injury in youths under 17 years old is almost nonexistent. This may have to do with the small number of participants in this age group. Virtually all fatalities and serious central nervous system damage (acute or chronic) have been in higher-level boxing.[1]

From a medical standpoint, participation in boxing cannot be recommended for any age group. If children participate, adequate head protection, good supervision, and early intervention at the slightest sign of injury is mandatory. It is important to note that the American Academy of Pediatrics has taken a position against boxing for children and young adults. They state "children and young adults should be encouraged to participate in sports in which intentional head injury is not the primary objective of the sport."[60]

Soccer

Soccer is the most widely played team sport in the world. No deaths from head or spinal cord injury have been recorded, but concussions do occur.[1] Although head-to-head contact and falls are often responsible, "heading" the ball remains the riskiest activity. Bruce and associates[1] quoted an unpublished study by Roberts and Corsellis that described five cases of chronic encephalopathy from repeated heading of the ball. Coaches should not encourage heading until the children are old enough to receive instruction on proper techniques.

Soccer may be the safest contact sport for school-age children. With proper coaching and supervision, the incidence of severe central nervous system injury should be zero.[1]

Baseball

Baseball has a low incidence of severe central nervous system injury. No deaths have been reported from head or spinal cord injury. The few reports of neurologic injury document concussions from impact by a ball or bat.[1] The use of helmets by batters is mandatory.

Bicycling

Every year 1300 people die in bicycle accidents.[61] Brain injuries cause 75% of both fatalities and disabling injuries in bicycle accidents.

McDermott and Klug[62] compared injuries caused by bicycles with those caused by motorcycles. Motorcyclists sustained more severe injuries to the body but bicyclists sustained more frequent and severe head injuries. This was attributed to the use of helmets by motorcyclists. Similar findings were demonstrated by Waters[63] and by Simpson and associates.[64] The latter recommended the use of helmets for cyclists and the establishment of cycle lanes to separate bicyclists from motor vehicles.

The use of helmets in contact sports has dramatically decreased the incidence of serious brain injury. The focus for injury prevention in bicycling, therefore, is on the use of helmets. Although helmet use is controversial,[2,65] all authors agree that their regular use would significantly decrease the number of serious head injuries incurred in recreational bicycling. An effective helmet should absorb the energy of the crash, distribute forces over the helmet rather than the head, and provide protection against sharp objects.[11,66]

Summary

Child athletes may be less susceptible to spinal cord injury than their older counterparts. Whether this results from an intrinsic property of the immature spine and spinal cord, the decreased weight and speed of the participants, or a lack of data on the number of athletes at risk is unknown.

It is unlikely that significant head and spinal cord injuries will ever be eliminated in sports. The nature of the activities requires that the head and spine be placed at risk. Changes in equipment, however, have greatly decreased the incidence of severe brain injury. Concomitant with this has been an increase in spinal injury, probably because the increased confidence of the participant results in greater use of the head for contact purposes. Rule changes designed to eliminate the use of the head as a battering ram have decreased the risk of serious injury in many sports. Better education, supervision, and coaching may decrease the number of injuries in diving, boxing, wrestling, trampolining, and gymnastics but will be unable to make these sports completely safe.

References

1. Bruce DA, Schut L, Sutton LN: Brain and cervical spine injuries occurring during organized sports activities in children and adolescents. *Primary Care* 1984;11:175-194.
2. Ciastko AR: Why I have difficulty being enthusiastic about recommending that children wear helmets on bicycles, letter. *Pediatrics* 1987;79:487-488.
3. Kalsbeek WD, McLaurin RL, Harris BS III, et al: The National Head and Spinal Cord Injury Survey: Major findings. *J Neurosurg* 1980;53(suppl):S19-S31.
4. Tator CH, Edmonds VE: Acute spinal cord injury: Analysis of epidemiologic factors. *Can J Surg* 1979;22:575-578.
5. Yngve DA, Harris WP, Herndon WA, et al: Spinal cord injury without osseous spine fracture. *J Pediatr Orthop* 1988;8:153-159.
6. Young JS, Burns PE, Bowen AM, et al: *Spinal Cord Injury Statistics: Experience of the Regional Spinal Cord Injury Systems.* Phoenix, Good Samaritan Medical Center, 1982.
7. Torg JS, Vegso JJ, Sennett B, et al: The National Football Head and Neck Injury Registry: 14-year report on cervical quadriplegia, 1971 through 1984. *JAMA* 1985;254:3439-3443.
8. Albright JP, Moses JM, Feldick HG, et al: Nonfatal cervical spine injuries in interscholastic football. *JAMA* 1976;236:1243-1245.
9. Torg JS, Quedenfeld TC, Burstein A, et al: National Football Head and Neck Injury: Registry Report on cervical quadriplegia, 1971 to 1975. *Am J Sports Med* 1979;7:127-132.
10. Torg JS, Truex R JR, Quedenfeld TC, et al: The National Football Head and Neck Injury Registry: Report and conclusions 1978. *JAMA* 1979;274:1477-1479.
11. Virgin H: Cineradiographic study of football helmets and the cervical spine. *Am J Sports Med* 1980;8:310-317.
12. Bauze RJ, Ardran GM: Experimental production of forward dislocation in the human cervical spine. *J Bone Joint Surg* 1978;60B:239-245.
13. Burstein AH, Otis JC, Torg JS: Mechanisms and pathomechanics of athletic injuries to the cervical spine, in Torg JS (ed): *Athletic Injuries to the Head, Neck, and Face.* Philadelphia, Lea & Febiger, 1982, pp 139-154.

14. Torg JS: Epidemiology, pathomechanics, and prevention of athletic injuries to the cervical spine. *Med Sci Sports Exerc* 1985;17:295-303.

15. Alexander MJ: Biomechanical aspects of lumbar spine injuries in athletes: A review. *Can J Appl Sport Sci* 1985;10:1-20.

16. Ferguson RJ, McMaster JH, Stanitski CL: Low back pain in college football linemen. *J Sports Med* 1974;2:63-69.

17. McCarroll JR, Miller JM, Ritter MA: Lumbar spondylolysis and spondylolisthesis in college football players: A prospective study. *Am J Sports Med* 1986;14:404-406.

18. Cantu RC: Lumbar spine injuries, in Cantu RC (ed): *The Exercising Adult*. Lexington, Massachusetts, Collamore Press, 1982, pp 143-157.

19. Burke DC: Spinal cord injuries from water sports. *Med J Aust* 1972;2:1190-1194.

20. Kewalramani LS, Orth MS, Taylor RG: Injuries to the cervical spine from diving accidents. *J Trauma* 1975;15:130-142.

21. Tator CH, Edmonds VE, New ML: Diving: A frequent and potentially preventable cause of spinal cord injury. *Can Med Assoc J* 1981;124:1323-1324.

22. Shields CL, Fox JM, Stauffer ES: Cervical cord injuries in sports. *Phys Sportsmed* 1978;6:71-76.

23. Albrand OW, Walter J: Underwater deceleration curves in relation to injuries from diving. *Surg Neurol* 1975;4:461-464.

24. Centers for Disease Control: Diving-associated spinal cord injuries during drought conditions: Wisconsin, 1988. *MMWR* 1988;37:453-454.

25. Zimmerman HM: Accident experience with trampolines. *Res Q* 1946;27:452-455.

26. Ellis WG, Green D, Holzaepfel NR, et al: The trampoline and serious neurological injuries: A report of five cases. *JAMA* 1960;174:1673-1676.

27. Torg JS, Das M: Trampoline-related quadriplegia: Review of the literature and reflections on the American Academy of Pediatrics position statement. *Pediatrics* 1984;74:804-812.

28. Frykman G, Hilding S: Hopp pa studsmatta kan orsaka allvarliga skador. *Lakartidningen* 1970;67:5862-5864.

29. Hammer A, Schwartzbach AL, Darre E, et al: Svaere neurologiske skader som folge af tramplinspring. *Ugeskr Laeger* 1981;143:2970-2974.

30. Steinbruck JK, Paeslack V: Trampolinspringen: Ein gefahrlicher Sport? Verletzungsanalysen und prophylaktische Massnahmen. *Munch Med Wochenschr* 1978;120:985-988.

31. Witthaut H: Verletzungen beim Trampolinturnen. *Monatschr Unfallheilkd* 1969;72:25-29.

32. Hage P: Trampolines: An "attractive nuisance." *Phys Sportsmed* 1970;10:118-122.

33. Rapp GF, Nicely PG: Trampoline injuries. *Am J Sports Med* 1978;6:260-271.

34. Rapp GF: Problems with the trampoline: II. Safety suggestions for trampoline use. *Pediatr Ann* 1978;7:730-731.

35. Clarke KS: A survey of sports-related spinal cord injuries in schools and colleges, 1973-1975. *J Safety Res* 1977;9:140-147.

36. American Academy of Pediatrics, Committee on Accident and Poison Prevention: Trampolines. Evanston, American Academy of Pediatrics, 1977.

37. Christensen C, Clarke KS: *Fourth Annual Gymnastic Catastrophic Injury Report, 1981-82*. Urbana-Champaign, University of Illinois, 1982.

38. American Academy of Pediatrics, Committee on Accident and Poison Prevention and Committee on Pediatric Aspects of Physical Fitness, Recreation, and Sports: Trampolines II. *Pediatrics* 1981;67:438.

39. Hooper J: Gymnastic injuries. *Aust Fam Physician* 1984;13:508-509.

40. Jackson DW, Wiltse LL, Cirincoine RJ: Spondylolysis in the female gymnast. *Clin Orthop* 1976;117:68-73.

41. Garrick JG, Requa RK: Epidemiology of women's gymnastics injuries. *Am J Sports Med* 1980;8:261-264.

42. Fekete JF: Severe brain injury and death following minor hockey accidents: The effectiveness of the "safety helmets" of amateur hockey players. *Can Med Assoc J* 1968;99:1234-1239.

43. Feriencik K: Trends in ice hockey injuries: 1965 to 1977. *Phys Sportsmed* 1979;7:81-84.

44. Tator CH, Ekong CE, Rowed DW, et al: Spinal injuries due to hockey. *Can J Neurol Sci* 1984;11:34-41.

45. Tator CH, Edmonds VE: National survey of spinal injuries in hockey players. *Can Med Assoc J* 1981;124:1323-1324.

46. Gerberich SG, Finke R, Madden M, et al: An epidemiological study of high school ice hockey injuries. *Childs Nerv Syst* 1987;3:59-64.

47. Sim FH, Simonet WT, Melton LJ III, et al: Ice hockey injuries. *Am J Sports Med* 1987;15:30-40.

48. Bishop PJ, Norman RW, Wells R, et al: Changes in the centre of mass and moment of inertia of a headform induced by a hockey helmet and face shield. *Can J Appl Sport Sci* 1983;8:19-25.

49. Smith AW, Bishop PJ, Wells RP: Alterations in head dynamics with the addition of a hockey helmet and face shield under inertial loading. *Can J Appl Sport Sci* 1985;10:68-74.

50. Norman RW: Biomechanical evaluations of sports protective equipment. *Exerc Sport Sci Rev* 1983;11:232-274.

51. Scher AT: Vertex impact and cervical dislocation in rugby players. *S Afr Med J* 1981;59:227-228.

52. Burry HC, Gowland H: Cervical injury in rugby football: A New Zealand survey. *Br J Sports Med* 1981;15:56-59.

53. Taylor TK, Coolican MR: Spinal-cord injuries in Australian footballers, 1960-1985. *Med J Aust* 1987;147:112-118.

54. Davidson RM: Schoolboy rugby injuries, 1969-1986. *Med J Aust* 1987;147:119-120.

55. McCoy GF, Piggot J, Macafee AL, et al: Injuries of the cervical spine in schoolboy rugby football. *J Bone Joint Surg* 1984;66B:500-503.

56. Gonzales TA: Fatal injuries in competitive sports. *JAMA* 1951;146:1506-1511.

57. Leidholt JD: Spinal injuries in athletes: Be prepared. *Orthop Clin North Am* 1973;4:691-717.

58. Wu WQ, Lewis RC: Injuries of the cervical spine in high school wrestling. *Surg Neurol* 1985;23:143-147.

59. Brain damage in sport, editorial. *Lancet* 1976;1:401-402.

60. American Academy of Pediatrics, Committee on Sports Medicine: Particpation in boxing among children and young adults. *Pediatrics* 1984;74:311-312.

61. Metz SE: Bicycle helmet education project, letter. *Am J Dis Child* 1988;142:414-415.

62. McDermott FT, Klug GL: Head injury predominance: Pedal-cyclists vs. motor-cyclists. *Med J Aust* 1985;143:232-234.

63. Waters EA: Should pedal cyclists wear helmets? A comparison of head injuries sustained by pedal cyclists and motorcyclists in road traffic accidents. *Injury* 1986;17:372-375.

64. Simpson AHRW, Unwin PS, Nelson IW: Head injuries, helmets, cycle lanes, and cyclists. *Br Med J* 1988;296:116-117.

65. Weiss BD: Childhood bicycle injuries: What can we do? *Am J Dis Child* 1987;141:135-136.

66. McLean AJ: Neurotrauma on two wheels. *Aust NZ J Surg* 1985;55:425-426.

Chapter 18

Injuries to the Shoulder Girdle and Elbow

John F. Meyers, MD

Introduction

Injuries in the young athlete differ significantly from those in the adult. Open epiphyses and soft articular cartilage are vulnerable to injury in this age group. Repetitive trauma can lead to overuse syndromes and microfractures. It is important for those who treat young athletes to recognize patterns of injury that are both age-specific and sports-specific, to know which injuries allow a return to competition when successfully treated and which have a potential for long-term damage and to attempt to define the measures that might prevent injuries to young athletes.

Shoulder Injuries

Tibone[1] defined the differences between injuries to the shoulder girdle in children and those in adults. The joint capsule and the ligaments in a child are approximately two to five times as strong as the epiphyseal plate. An injury that would cause a torn ligament in an adult produces a fracture through the hypertrophic zone of the epiphysis in a child. Because radiographs are sometimes difficult to interpret in a growing child, it is important to recognize this difference and to look for fractures that involve the growth centers.

Clavicle   Injury to the sternoclavicular joint that would cause a dislocation in an adult causes an epiphyseal fracture in a child. The medial epiphysis closes at 22 years of age; before this time, epiphyseal fractures are more common than dislocations. Radiographs of the sternoclavicular joint are particularly difficult to evaluate. If the diagnosis is in doubt, a computed tomographic scan is helpful in defining the sternoclavicular joint. Because these fractures remodel, open treatment of the sternoclavicular dislocation is only indicated in a posterior irreducible dislocation that might injure the great vessels.

Acromioclavicular separations are rare before the age of 13 years. An apparent acromioclavicular separation in this age group is usually a fracture of the distal clavicular epiphysis with a tear of the coracoacromial ligament or a fracture through the subcoracoid epiphysis with the ligaments remaining intact. Closed treatment is also successful in this injury because of the remodeling potential of the bone in the growing child.

Cahill[2] described osteolysis of the distal clavicle in weightlifters. However, the youngest patient in his series was 19 years old. As weight training has become more popular in the training of younger athletes, this lesion is being seen in a younger population. Pain and swelling about the acromioclavicular joint usually are first noticed during bench presses or dips. Radiographs show a loss of subchondral bone and a bone scan shows increased activity in the distal clavicle. The etiology of osteolysis of the distal clavicle is unclear. An inflammatory process has been postulated, as has microfracture secondary to repeated stress. Treatment consists of altering the athlete's training techniques. If the hands are held closer together during the bench press, there is less shear on the distal clavicle and this exercise can be resumed. If this is not successful, bench presses should be avoided. Conservative treatment usually leads to resolution of symptoms and new bone formation in the distal clavicle. Cahill[2] reported successful treatment in recalcitrant cases by resection of the distal clavicle in the skeletally mature patient.

Glenohumeral Joint   Fractures of the proximal humeral epiphysis resulting from trauma are usually Salter I or Salter II fractures. These can be treated conservatively with good results regardless of the amount of displacement.[3] Surgical reduction is only indicated for tenting of the skin or vascular compromise. Rotational stresses placed on the young athlete's shoulder can result in damage to the physis. The entity described by Adams[4] as osteochondrosis of the proximal humeral physis is now called Little League shoulder. Cahill and associates[5] believe that it results from repetitive stress caused by rotatory torque during the cocking and acceleration phases or deceleration distraction forces during follow-through in pitching. These forces result in a stress fracture of the epiphyseal plate. Radiographs show widening of the epiphyseal line at first. Subsequently, there is metaphyseal and diaphyseal new bone formation secondary to periosteal stripping. This lesion heals with rest alone. Rest should be enforced until the symptoms subside because persistent stress could lead to displacement or rupture of the epiphyseal plate.

Glenohumeral Dislocation and Subluxation   The design of the shoulder joint allows for maximum freedom of movement. The shoulder relies on soft-tissue restraints, not its bony architecture, for stability. Because of this anatomic design the shoulder is the most frequently dislocated joint.

Perry[6] described the restraints to anterior dislocation of the shoulder. The relatively flat glenoid is retroverted approximately seven degrees.

The presence of the glenoid labrum increases the area of contact with the humeral head from one-third to three-fourths that of the humeral head. The anterior capsule is reinforced by a thickened area known as the anterior inferior glenohumeral ligament. The tendon of the subscapularis adds to anterior stability with the arm at the side. If abduction exceeds 90 degrees, the humeral head can pass anteriorly beneath the subscapularis tendon. McGlynn and Caspari[7] described the arthroscopic findings in the dislocated and subluxated shoulder. They found incompetence of the anterior inferior glenohumeral ligament and Hill-Sachs lesions or an indentation on the posterior aspect of the humeral head, caused by pressure from the anterior glenoid as the head slides anteriorly. In younger patients, this incompetence resulted from a tearing of the labrum from the glenoid anteriorly.

Long-term follow-up of dislocation of the shoulder[8,9] shows that recurrent dislocation is a problem in the younger patient. As many as 66% of dislocations in those under the age of 20 years may become recurrent, whereas few recurrent dislocations develop in patients over 40 years old. Simonet and Cofield[9] found that recurrent dislocations are a particular problem in young athletes. There is an 82% recurrence rate in this population. Treatment after reduction should consist of immobilization in internal rotation for three weeks and restriction from competition for six weeks. Although stability depends more on capsular integrity than on muscular strength, a complete rehabilitation program is recommended before return to competition because of the danger of injury to the weakened shoulder girdle.

Early results of arthroscopic treatment of recurrent dislocation of the shoulder are encouraging. An arthroscopic Bankart repair with sutures can be performed on those patients who have Bankart lesions. An arthroscopic capsular plication can be performed in patients without Bankart lesions and in whom the ligament was incompetent. One group had a 92% success rate after a two-year follow-up in a series of 40 cases.[10] Others reported less successful results using arthroscopic staples to plicate the anterior capsule.[11]

Posterior dislocations of the shoulder are rare. They constitute approximately 4% of all shoulder dislocations. Posterior subluxations of the shoulder are more common. In the series of Hawkins and associates,[12] the average age at onset of the instability was 16 years. Trauma was usually minor or absent in these patients. Voluntary subluxation can usually be exhibited by the patients when the arm is abducted and forward flexed with selective muscle contraction. This condition is symptomatic when the subluxation becomes unintentional. This group should be distinguished from those patients who have psychiatric disturbances and whose subluxations are willful and habitual. Treatment of posterior subluxation is difficult. Hawkins and associates reported a success rate of only 50% after surgical treatment. Norwood and Terry[13] also had a 50% success rate, but they believed that the prognosis was better if an initial traumatic episode caused the subluxation.

Pappas and associates[14] described functional instability caused by tears of the glenoid labrum. The torn labrum can become displaced in the joint much like a bucket-handle tear of the meniscus, causing locking and pain. These symptoms are usually reproducible by rotation of the arm in the fully forward flexed position. Arthroscopic evaluation clearly defines the abnormality, and labral tears can be resected arthroscopically. It is important to recognize that tears of the anteroinferior labrum are usually associated with instability and that this instability must be treated or symptoms will persist.

Impingement   Impingement of the supraspinatus tendon beneath the coracoacromial arch is common in athletes involved in swimming, throwing, and racket sports.[15,16] In swimmers the incidence of shoulder problems seems to increase with the ability of the swimmer. As many as 57% of championship swimmers have shoulder problems. The average age at onset in swimmers is 18 years.

Neer[17] clearly defined the cause of the impingement syndrome. The functional position of the shoulder is one of forward flexion and not abduction. In this position, the supraspinatus tendon and the long head of the biceps pass beneath the anterior edge and the undersurface of the acromion and the coracoclavicular and coracoacromial ligaments. Neer believes that impingement is more likely to develop in a patient with a prominent anterior acromion or abnormal inferior angulation. Impingement is a continuum and, if left untreated, progresses from stage I, with inflammation and swelling, through stage III, with eventual rotator cuff tears.

Nirschl[18] believes that the primary problem in the impingement syndrome lies in the rotator cuff tendons and not in the coracoacromial arch. Rotator cuff tendinitis is related to an intrinsic overload of the tendons. Pathologic changes in the tendon cause muscle weakness and imbalance and, eventually, upward migration of the humeral head. Impingement does occur, but as a secondary rather than a primary phenomenon. The rotator cuff stabilizes the humeral head against the glenoid when the deltoid acts in abduction and forward flexion. If the normal strength of the rotator cuff is lost, the humeral head migrates proximally as the deltoid contracts, causing impingement. Glousman[19] and Micheli[20] believe that impingement in the young athlete is often secondary to subtle instabilities of the shoulder. Progressive attenuation of the anterior static restraints of the shoulder allows a traction injury of the rotator cuff to occur. In this instance, primary treatment should be aimed at the instability rather than the secondary impingement. Physical signs may be subtle and arthroscopy is often necessary to define this instability.

Conservative treatment is usually successful in the young athlete with stage I impingement. Treatment should consist of rest, ice, and nonsteroidal anti-inflammatory medications. Rehabilitation should be designed to regain full range of motion of the shoulder and to strengthen the musculature of the rotator cuff. Changes in the training regimen and the technique of the athletic activity are often necessary to prevent recurrence. Successful surgical treatment, which consists of incision of the coracoacromial ligament, has been reported, but this operation should rarely be necessary if proper conservative care has been administered.[16,20]

Elbow Injuries

Injuries of the elbow occur primarily in throwing athletes and gymnasts. Although the injuries are often similar in baseball and gymnastics, their treatment and prognoses are different.

Baseball Injuries   Studies of Little League pitchers in Houston, TX,[21] and Eugene, OR,[22] have shown a 20% incidence of symptoms of elbow pain in 11- and 12-year-old pitchers. Radiographs showed abnormalities of the medial elbow in 28% and of the lateral elbow in 5%. Adams,[23] who examined pitchers in this age group in southern California, found a 45% incidence of elbow pain and a 100% incidence of radiographic changes. He attributed this to the much longer baseball season in the more temperate climate. The problem of elbow pain seems to increase with age and exposure. Grana and Rashkin[24] found a 58% incidence of elbow pain in high-school pitchers (average age, 17 years). Fifty-six percent had radiographic abnormalities and 4% had loose bodies.

The cause of elbow problems in the throwing athlete can be characterized in one word—valgus. The valgus forces generated during the acceleration phase of pitching cause distraction on the medial side of the elbow and compression on the lateral side. Abnormalities on the medial side vary with the age of the athlete. In the child, traction forces result in hypertrophy of the medial epicondyle, microtears of the flexor pronator group, and, often, fragmentation of the epicondylar apophysis. During adolescence, increased muscular strength can cause avulsion fractures through the epiphysis. If these fractures are displaced, open reduction and internal fixation is indicated. After closure of the epiphysis at 15 years of age,[25] avulsion of a fragment of bone, rather than of the entire apophysis, is usual. A small and displaced fragment is often associated with a tear of the anterior band of the medial collateral ligament. A gravity abduction stress radiograph is helpful in defining the instability secondary to tearing of the medial collateral ligament. Ligament repair should be undertaken if this test is positive.

Repetitive valgus stress can cause traction, stretching, and inflammation of the ulnar nerve as it passes behind the medial epicondyle. The nerve can also be compressed by fibers of the flexor carpi ulnaris as it enters the muscle. If conservative treatment does not alleviate the symptoms, surgical exploration of the nerve is indicated. Anterior transposition may be necessary.

Lateral compression generated by valgus stress may lead to bony changes of osteochondritis dissecans of the capitellum and the radial head. Osteochondritis dissecans occurs in those 13 to 17 years old. This entity should not be confused with Panner's disease.[26] Panner's disease occurs before the age of 11 years and is a benign, self-limited process characterized by fragmentation of the entire ossific center of the capitellum. It requires only conservative care. Loose bodies are not formed in Panner's disease. Osteochondritis dissecans differs from Panner's disease in that it occurs in adolescents and consists of a localized area of avascular necrosis on the anterolateral aspect of the capitellum. It is often complicated by breakdown of bone and articular cartilage with subsequent formation of loose bodies in the elbow. Haraldson[27] described how the anatomic arrangement of the blood vessels that supply the capitellum places it at risk. Before epiphyseal closure, the only blood supply to the epiphysis is through one or two large blood vessels that enter the epiphysis from its posterior aspect. No vessels cross the epiphyseal plate from the metaphysis. After epiphyseal closure at age 19, there are anastomoses among the metaphyseal, diaphyseal, and capitellar vessels.

McManama and associates[28] reported excellent results with surgical treatment of osteochondritis dissecans. Eighty-six percent of their athletes returned to organized athletics without restrictions. Their surgical treatment consisted of removal of loose bodies, excision of capitellar lesions, and curettage of the base. They do not recommend bone grafting and pinning of loose fragments. Others have reported less favorable results after surgical treatment.[29]

Posterior elbow problems, although less common, may also occur in the throwing athlete. As the elbow is rapidly extended from a flexed position, forceful contraction of the triceps may result in triceps tendinitis. Repeated traction on the olecranon epiphysis by the triceps tendon is thought to be responsible for a traction-type apophysitis of the olecranon similar to that seen on the medial epicondyle. Repetitive trauma can lead to actual nonunion of the epiphysis. Excellent results have been reported with open reduction and bone graft of this nonunion.[30]

The long-term effects of pitching on the athlete growing into adulthood were described by Jobe and Moynes.[31] Reactive spurs are seen on the medial epicondyle. Spurs form on the medial aspect of the olecranon from repetitive contact with the medial aspect of the olecranon fossa. This can result in the formation of loose bodies in the posterior compartment of the elbow. Stretching, causing incompetence of the anterior band of the ulnar collateral ligament and medial instability, is also a common problem in the adult athlete.

Preventing these throwing injuries requires proper technique and limited exposure to throwing. Pappas[32] believes that the forces acting on the elbow vary with different types of pitches. Throwing a curve ball causes more difficulties on the medial aspect of the elbow. This is secondary to the sudden contractive forces of the wrist and finger flexors when the arm is maintained in supination. Throwing a fast ball generates more force across the radiocapitellar joint. Albright and associates[33] believe that the position of the elbow relative to the shoulder at the time of ball release is the most important factor in generating forces across the elbow. Among pitchers who used a sidearm delivery 74% reported elbow problems, whereas only 27% of the pitchers who used a vertical delivery had elbow pain. Limiting the number of innings pitched and the number of pitches thrown by Little Leaguers has significantly decreased elbow symptoms.[34]

Gymnastics Snook[35] was the first to point out the high incidence of injuries in competitive gymnastics. The elbow is quite vulnerable in gymnastics because it is converted from a nonweightbearing to a weightbearing joint. Fractures and dislocations of the elbow are the most common serious gymnastic injury of the upper extremity.[36] Standard fracture care is indicated, but motion should be reinstituted as early as possible. Triceps tendinitis is a frequent complaint.[37] The olecranon and triceps tendon become inflamed because the elbow is locked into hyperextension during weightbearing. Standard conservative treatment, as well as strengthening of the biceps so that the olecranon need not be locked into hyperflexion to maintain weightbearing, is the treatment of choice.

The valgus-carrying angle of the elbow during weightbearing subjects it to the same pathologic conditions that occur in pitchers.[38] Traction injuries to the medial elbow occur, as do compression injuries of the lateral elbow. Osteochondritis dissecans of the elbow seems to be a more serious problem in the gymnast than in the throwing athlete. Singer and Roy[39] were able to return four out of five high-performance female gymnasts with osteochondritis dissecans to competition after conservative and surgical treatment. However, the results deteriorated over time, and only one gymnast remains in competition. Jackson and associates[40] were unsuccessful in returning any of their series of 12 top-level gymnasts to their former competitive levels. They emphasized that gymnasts with elbow pain and loss of extension must undergo comprehensive study. Only half of their patients had radiographic abnormalities, but all had positive findings on bone scan and magnetic resonance imaging.

Early recognition and treatment remains a challenge in this disease. Perhaps the more frequent use of bone scans and magnetic resonance imaging will permit treatment before the disease becomes well established.

References

1. Tibone JE: Shoulder problems of adolescents. *Clin Sports Med* 1983;2:423-426.
2. Cahill BR: Osteolysis of the distal part of the clavicle in male athletes. *J Bone Joint Surg* 1982:64A:1053-1058.
3. Baxter MP, Wiley JJ: Fractures of the proximal humeral epiphysis: Their influence on humeral growth. *J Bone Joint Surg* 1986;68B:570-573.
4. Adams JE: Little League shoulder: Osteochondrosis of the proximal humeral epiphysis in boy baseball pitchers. *Calif Med* 1966;105:22-25.
5. Cahill BR, Tullos HS, Fain RH: Little League shoulder. *J Sports Med* 1974;2:150-152.
6. Perry J: Anatomy and biomechanics of the shoulder in throwing, swimming, gymnastics, and tennis. *Clin Sports Med* 1983;2:247-270.
7. McGlynn FJ, Caspari RB: Arthroscopic findings in the subluxating shoulder. *ClinOrthop* 1984;183:173-178.
8. Hovelius L: Anterior dislocation of the shoulder in teenagers and young adults: Five-year prognosis. *J Bone Joint Surg* 1987;69A:393-399.

9. Simonet WT, Cofield RH: Prognosis in anterior shoulder dislocation. *Am J Sports Med* 1984;12:19-24.

10. Caspari RB, Savoie FH, Meyers JF, et al: Arthroscopic management of the unstable shoulder. Presented at the annual meeting of the American Academy of Orthopaedic Surgeons, Feb 14, 1989.

11. Richardson AB: Arthroscopic stapling for treatment of anterior shoulder instability. Presented at the Eleventh International Seminar on Operative Arthroscopy, Oct 19, 1989.

12. Hawkins RJ, Koppert G, Johnston G: Recurrent posterior instability (subluxation) of the shoulder. *J Bone Joint Surg* 1984;66A:169-174.

13. Norwood LA, Terry GC: Shoulder posterior subluxation. *Am J Sports Med* 1984;12:25-30.

14. Pappas AM, Goss TP, Kleinman PK: Symptomatic shoulder instability due to lesions of the glenoid labrum. *Am J Sports Med* 1983;11:279-288.

15. Richardson AB, Jobe FW, Collins HR: The shoulder in competitive swimming. *Am J Sports Med* 1980;8:159-163.

16. Kennedy JC, Hawkins R, Krissoff WB: Orthopaedic manifestations of swimming. *Am J Sports Med* 1978;6:309-322.

17. Neer CS II: Anterior acromioplasty for the chronic impingement syndrome in the shoulder: A preliminary report. *J Bone Joint Surg* 1972;54A:41-50.

18. Nirschl RP: Shoulder tendinitis, in Pettrone FA (ed): American Academy of Orthopaedic Surgeons *Symposium on Upper Extremity Injuries in Athletes*. St. Louis, CV Mosby, 1986, ch 28.

19. Glousman R: The relationship of instability to rotator cuff damage: Conservative and surgical repair. Presented at the interim meeting of the American Orthopedic Society for Sports Medicine, Jan 7, 1988.

20. Micheli LJ: Overuse injuries in children's sports: The growth factor. *Orthop Clin North Am* 1983;14:337-360.

21. Gugenheim JJ Jr, Stanley RF, Woods GW, et al: Little League survey: The Houston study. *Am J Sports Med* 1976;4:189-200.

22. Larson RL, Singer KM, Bergstrom R, et al: Little League survey: The Eugene study. *Am J Sports Med* 1976;4:201-209.

23. Adams JE: Injuries to the throwing arm: A study of traumatic changes in the elbow joints of boy baseball players. *Cal Med* 1975;3:25-34.

24. Grana WA, Rashkin A: Pitcher's elbow in adolescents. *Am J Sports Med* 1980;8:333-336.

25. Woods GW, Tullos HS: Elbow instability and medial epicondyle fractures. *Am J Sports Med* 1977;5:23-30.

26. Panner HJ: An affection of the capitulum humeri resembling Calve-Perthes' disease of the hip. *Acta Radiol* 1927;8:617-618.

27. Haraldson S: On osteochondrosis deformans juvenilis capituli humeri including investigation of intra-osseous vasculature in distal humerus. *Acta Orthop Scand* 1959;38(suppl):1-232.

28. McManama GB Jr, Micheli LJ, Berry MV, et al: The surgical treatment of osteochondritis of the capitellum. *Am J Sports Med* 1985:13:11-21.

29. Tivnon MC, Anzel SH, Waugh TR: Surgical management of osteochondritis dissecans of the capitellum. *Am J Sports Med* 1976;4:121-128.

30. Pavlov H, Torg JS, Jacobs B, et al: Nonunion of olecranon epiphysis: Two cases in adolescent baseball pitchers. *AJR* 1981;136:819-820.

31. Jobe FW, Moynes DR: Delineation of diagnostic criteria and a rehabilitation program for rotator cuff injuries. *Am J Sports Med* 1982;10:336-339.

32. Pappas AM: Elbow problems associated with baseball during childhood and adolescence. *Clin Orthop* 1982;164:30-41.

33. Albright JA, Jokl P, Shaw R, et al: Clinical study of baseball pitchers: Correlation of injury to the throwing arm with method of delivery. *Am J Sports Med* 1978;6:15-21.

34. Torg JS, Pollack H, Sweterlisch P: The effect of competitive pitching on the shoulders and elbows of preadolescent baseball players. *Pediatrics* 1972;49:267-272.

35. Snook GA: Injuries in women's gymnastics. A 5-year study. *Am J Sports Med* 1979;7:242-244.

36. Priest JD, Weise DJ: Elbow injury in women's gymnastics. *Am J Sports Med* 1981;9:288-295.

37. Aronen JG: Problems of the upper extremity in gymnastics. *Clin Sports Med* 1985;4:61-71.

38. Goldberg MJ: Gymnastic injuries. *Orthop Clin North Am* 1980;11:717-726.

39. Singer KM, Roy SP: Osteochondrosis of the humeral capitellum. *Am J Sports Med* 1984;12:351-360.

40. Jackson DW, Runion PR, Morrison DS, et al: Osteochondritis dissecans in the female gymnast's elbow. Presented at the meeting of the Arthroscopy Association of North America, Washington, DC, March 1988.

Chapter 19

Injuries to the Hand and Wrist

Carlos A. Garcia-Moral, MD

Injuries to the hand and wrist are common and may affect the athlete's ability to compete. Impaired hand functioning may even influence the athlete's future choice of career. Most injuries to the athlete's hand are closed injuries to the finger and wrist that affect primarily the muscle-tendon units, ligamentous injuries to the joints, neurovascular disturbances, fractures, and dislocations.

Epidemiology

Athletic participation enhances the development and maintenance of physical and mental fitness and health. The direct and indirect risks of athletic competition include injuries. Several factors influence the type, location, and extent of injuries sustained by the young athlete. These factors may be related to the athlete, the activity, or environmental factors.[1]

Factors related to the athlete include age, sex, personal habits, experience, level of fitness, and general health. The activity factors include the number of participants, the technique, the frequency and duration of participation, and practice sessions. Environmental factors include location, weather conditions, playing surface, and equipment.

Little information is available on the rate or severity of injuries in children before they enter high school.[2,3,4,5] Some studies have shown that the incidence of injury depends on the age of the children.[2,3,6] Children under 12 years old appear to have a lower incidence of injury.

Although there may be discrepancies in the reported incidences of sports-related injuries, the risk of significant injury with permanent functional impairment does exist. The most frequent site of sports-related injuries is the hand,[7] and their incidence varies with the sport and position of the player in the team during participation.[8,9,10] A large number of sport injuries that result in a permanent functional impairment at a later time in the athlete's life remain unknown to epidemiologists.

Ligament Injuries

In children with open physes, the collateral ligaments of the metacarpophalangeal joints are attached to the epiphyses of the proximal pha-

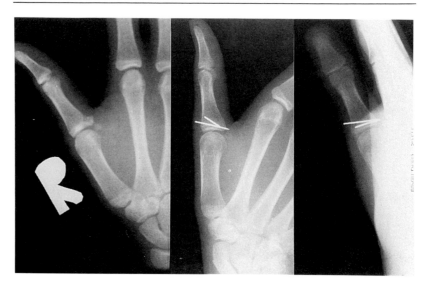

Fig. 1 *Type III Salter-Harris fracture of the proximal phalanx in a 16-year-old, treated with open reduction and internal fixation.*

lanx and metacarpal. The accessory collateral ligament extends proximally and crosses the growth plate to insert into the metaphysis of the metacarpal. The collateral ligaments of the proximal and distal interphalangeal joints have a deep portion that inserts into the epiphysis and more superficial fibers that extend to the metaphysis and blend with the periosteum of the phalanges.[11] Injury to these ligaments is uncommon in the skeletally immature athlete because they are much stronger relative to the physis.

Collateral Ligament Injuries
Thumb An injury to the ulnar collateral ligament of the thumb at the metacarpophalangeal joint is traditionally referred to as "gamekeeper's thumb."[12] Although this injury is common in skeletally mature athletes who participate in football, baseball, wrestling, and skiing, it is uncommon in young athletes. The mechanism of injury is usually forcible abduction or a combination of abduction and hyperextension of the joint. In the young athlete, the serious injury is damage to the physis of the proximal phalanx, and usually is a Type III Salter-Harris epiphyseal injury. These intra-articular fractures almost always require open reduction and internal fixation. (Fig. 1)

In older athletes, complete disruptions of the collateral ligament of the thumb's metacarpophalangeal joint or intra-articular avulsion fractures are managed by early surgical repair.[13] The ulnar collateral ligament is usually avulsed from its insertion in the proximal phalanx and in 75% of the cases there is a Stener lesion present at surgery.[14]

Partial tears without joint instability can be satisfactorily managed by thumb spica cast immobilization for four to six weeks, followed by a period of protected splinting or thumb taping during sport activities.

Proximal Interphalangeal Joint Most injuries to the small joints of the fingers are caused by partial tears of the ligamentous structures without compromise of joint stability. These occur in skeletally mature individuals. Most investigators believe that partial tears respond favorably to immobilization of the joint in extension for three weeks, followed by protective "buddy" splinting of the adjacent finger.[15]

Traumatic Tendon Ruptures

These injuries are also uncommon in the young athlete. However, three injuries that deserve mention are loss of extensor continuity at the proximal, distal interphalangeal joint and rupture of the flexor profundus tendon.

Other tendon injuries are uncommon and include longitudinal tears of the sagittal band, avulsion of the flexor digitorum sublimis and dislocation of the extensor carpi ulnaris tendon.

Mallet Finger Deformity Longitudinal force applied to the distal phalanx of a finger can produce an extensor tendon rupture, avulsion fracture, or fracture subluxation of the distal interphalangeal joint.

Surgery is rarely indicated for a mallet finger injury except in open tendon lacerations and in epiphyseal fractures that cause avulsion of the nail from the matrix and require surgical debridement and reduction of the nail under the eponychial fold with reduction of the fracture. (Fig. 2)

Epiphyseal plate injuries are usually Salter-Harris Type II or III.[16] The growth plate of the distal phalanx usually remains open until age 15. Epiphyseal injuries in the young child usually require a period of immobilization with splinting for as long as six weeks.

In all other types of mallet finger deformity, the best treatment is splinting with the distal interphalangeal joint in 0 degrees of extension for eight weeks followed by progressive and gentle exercises until motion has reached 35 degrees of flexion and full extension. The splint can then be discontinued.

Whether an athlete with this injury should participate in sports depends on the sport and its requirements; a compliant athlete can compete with an immobilization splint.

Avulsion of the Flexor Digitorum Profundus Tendon Avulsion of the insertion of the flexor tendon in the terminal phalanx is a fairly common injury. Flexor tendon injuries classically occur in rugby or football when a defensive player grabs the jersey of an opponent and the flexor tendon is pulled from its insertion with great force. This injury usually occurs in the ring finger.

The diagnosis is initially often overlooked.[17,18] The symptoms in-

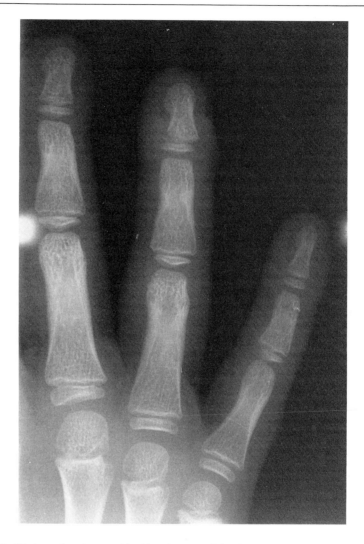

Fig. 2 *AP view of an 8-year-old with a fracture of the distal phalanx of the ring finger and avulsion of the nail from its matrix.*

clude pain and marked swelling of the finger or palm of the hand and inability to flex the distal phalanx. After the diagnosis is made, the athlete's hand must be protected until a treatment decision is reached. The treatment of choice in an acute injury is prompt surgical repair; this generally produces the best result. There are reports[19,20] of this type of intra-articular fracture associated with the simultaneous avulsion of the flexor digitorum profundus tendon. Four weeks after the injury, primary reattachment of the tendon in the distal phalanx may be difficult and alternative procedures, such as tenodesis (especially for the ring and small fingers)[21] or arthrodesis (for the index and middle fingers), should be considered.

Recurrent Dislocation of the Extensor Carpi Ulnaris Tendon   The extensor carpi ulnaris tendon inserts into the base of the fifth metacarpal on the ulnar aspect of the wrist and occupies the six dorsal extensor compartments under the extensor retinaculum. Recurrent dislocation of the extensor carpi ulnaris tendon is caused by disruption or stretching of the tendon sheath at the level of the distal ulna.[22]

Sports activities that require sudden supination, flexion, and ulnar deviation of the wrist may produce disruption or stretching of the fibrous tunnel of the extensor carpi ulnaris tendon, leading to recurrent dislocation. Golf, baseball, and racket sports are the main offenders. The diagnosis is not difficult; there is a painful snapping sensation in the ulnar aspect of the wrist on supination, flexion, and ulnar deviation of the wrist. This injury is sometimes associated with fractures of the ulnar styloid.

Conservative treatment with immobilization or a temporary decrease in activity is usually unsuccessful, and surgical reconstruction of the dorsal extensor compartment is the procedure of choice for chronic recurrent dislocation.

Longitudinal Tears of the Extensor Tendon   This uncommon injury is usually the result of direct trauma to the extensor mechanism while the metacarpophalangeal joint is being flexed. The extensor tendon is ruptured by longitudinal tears at the sagittal bands or between the extensor digitorum communis and extensor indicis proprius in the index finger. Usually these tears occur at the level of the metacarpophalangeal joints.

Clinically, there is recurrent pain and swelling of the metacarpophalangeal joint. Occasionally a bursa is present. Subluxation of the extensor tendon to one side of the metacarpal head can be seen on examination. Surgical repair of the longitudinal defect is the procedure of choice.[16] This type of injury occurs most often in boxers.[9]

Growth Center Injuries

Growth center injury in the hand represents a diagnostic and treatment challenge. In the young athlete, the unique configuration of the growth center and the physiologic demands placed on it in sports make injuries to the hand different from those in older athletes. In children there is an increased incidence of fractures in the early years, the time at which children start sport activities. Epiphyseal fractures or injuries represent 34% of all fractures in young patients.[23]

The growth plates in the fingers are located proximally; they are located distally in metacarpals II through V and proximally in metacarpal I. They appear in the fingers at about 3 years of age and have

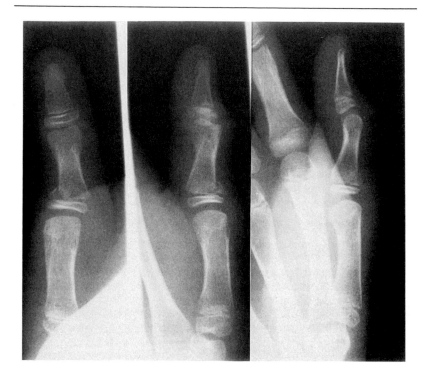

Fig. 3 *A 13-year-old goalie of a soccer team sustained this typical Type II fracture of the thumb.*

fused by 18 years of age. The Salter-Harris classification of epiphyseal fractures is the most commonly used.[24]

A Salter-Harris I fracture involves separation of the epiphysis and diaphysis and usually occurs in early childhood. The mechanism of this type of injury is pure shear and the prognosis is good.

A Salter-Harris II includes a wedge of the metaphyseal bone attached to the epiphysis. (Fig. 3) This injury usually occurs after the age of ten years. The mechanism of injury is by shear or avulsion with an angular force. This represents the most common type of epiphyseal injury in fractures of the hand—78.7%. Of this type, the proximal phalanx was involved in 69%, the middle phalanx in 25%, and the metacarpal and distal phalanx[24] 8% of the time in each case.

Type III fractures extend through the physis and across the epiphysis into the joint. Again, this type of injury occurs after the age of ten and the mechanism of injury is from an intra-articular avulsion force. The prognosis can be poor unless early accurate reduction can be obtained, as commonly seen in the thumb. (Fig. 1)

A Salter-Harris IV fracture extends across both the epiphysis and the metaphysis and can occur at any age; however, it is extremely rare in the hand. The mechanism of injury is compression loading of a portion of the articular surface. The prognosis of this fracture is poor without an anatomic alignment.

A Salter-Harris V fracture involves crushing of the growth plate; this can also occur at any age and is extremely rare in the hand. The mechanism of injury is severe axial loading. The prognosis is poor because of the higher incidence of growth disturbance. (Fig. 4)

Epiphyseal injuries of the middle phalanx are rare. The collateral ligaments at the interphalangeal joints extend beyond the growth plate and blend with the periosteum of the metaphysis, providing better stability than at the metacarpophalangeal joints. Clinical alignment and rotation should be restored and the finger supported between the adjacent digits in a position between 10 degrees and full extension.

Salter-Harris III fractures also occur at the level of the proximal interphalangeal joint with the dorsal lip of the epiphysis avulsed by the central slip of the extensor tendon. These fractures require anatomic reduction of the dorsal epiphyseal fragment. Open reduction may be necessary to reduce and maintain this type of fracture.

Fractures of the proximal phalanx are probably among the most common epiphyseal injuries in the fingers. The most common is the Salter-Harris II fracture that results from forced rotation and angulation. It usually involves the index, ring, and little fingers. Angulatory deformities of more than 20 degrees are unacceptable and manipulation and reduction, with the patient under anesthesia, usually re-establishes the normal anatomic configuration of the proximal phalanx. Any rotation deformity is unacceptable because it will not remodel.

Salter-Harris III fractures of the thumb are common and mirror the avulsion of the ulnar or radial collateral ligaments in adults. These injuries usually involve small fragments and heal adequately with immobilization with no loss of stability; however, if the fragment is large and a significant portion of the joint is involved, open reduction and internal fixation may be indicated.

Epiphyseal injuries of the metacarpals usually occur in older children and are the result of a direct longitudinal force applied to the flexed metacarpophalangeal joints. Salter-Harris II fractures of the metacarpals, with a metaphyseal fracture proximal to the physis, are more common. These are the counterparts of boxer's fractures in adults. Remodeling of the volar angulation is expected in the young athlete. Angulation of 50 degrees is acceptable in the ring and little fingers; no more than 30 degrees of angulation is acceptable in the index and middle fingers. Again, rotational malalignment is unacceptable.

Bennett's fracture is uncommon in children, forming only 2% of first metacarpal fractures, but it accounts for about one-third of such fractures in adults.

The goal of treatment is accurate anatomic restoration of the articular surface. Closed treatment with percutaneous K-wire fixation, open reduction with percutaneous K-wire fixation, or open reduction and internal fixation through a volar approach may be needed.

Immobilization is maintained for as long as six weeks, after which the K-wires are removed and a program of active range-of-motion and

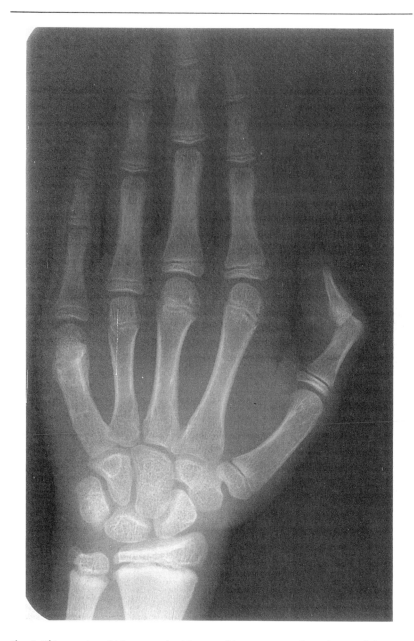

Fig. 4 *This rare type V fracture of a 13-year-old was sustained in a boxing fight. Note the early closure of the epiphysis.*

strengthening exercises is begun. Thumb splinting is continued for an additional six weeks.

Wrist Injuries

Fractures and ligamentous injuries of the carpal bones in children are less common than in adults.

At the time of birth none of the ossification centers of the carpal bones are present. The sequence of onset of the bone growth centers of the carpus begins with the capitate at about age three[26] for boys and girls and concludes with the pisiform at age eight for boys and ten for girls. The sequence of onset of carpal ossification begins with the capitate and continues with hamate, triquetrum, lunate, scaphoid, trapezoid, trapezium, and pisiform. This sequence may vary between the scaphoid, trapezoid and trapezium. The completion of ossification of the carpal is reached by 13.4 years old in girls and by 15.1 years old in boys.[25]

The scaphoid is the most common fracture of the carpal bone in children and the majority of injuries occur when the child is over ten years old.[26,27] The onset of the ossification center of the scaphoid appears by age five and expands eccentrically until ossification is completed.

The mechanism of injury is an axial load to the wrist with the hand in dorsiflexion. In the younger child, the mechanism of injury is usually a severe direct trauma, associated with other fractures. In approximately 49% and 52% of children, scaphoid fractures occur at the level of the distal third. Scaphoid fractures in children usually heal with prompt diagnosis at the time of injury and thumb spica cast immobilization.[26,28-32]

Although scaphoid nonunion in children has been reported by several authors,[29-31,33] it is rare and is generally the result of inadequate initial diagnosis or neglected treatment. The existence of multicenters of ossification in the scaphoid remains unclear.[34] Fractures of other carpal bones are very uncommon. Capitate fractures[35-37] and triquetrum have been reported in children.[38]

Posttraumatic carpal instability has been reported by Gerard[39] in a seven-year-old girl who fell from a table at the age of three months. Proximal migration of the capitate in the proximal carpal row was noted on anteroposterior roentgenograms.

Fracture dislocation of the carpus is also extremely rare in children but has been reported by Peiro[41] and others.

References

1. Maylack FH: Epidemiology of tennis, squash, and racquetball injuries. *Clin in Sports Med* 1988;7:233-243.
2. Nilsson S, Asbjorn R: Soccer injuries in adolescents. *Am J Sports Med* 1978; 6:358-361.

3. Sullivan JA, Gross RH, Grana WA, et al: Evaluation of injuries in youth soccer. *Am J Sports Med* 1980;8:325-327.
4. Larson RL, Singer KM, Bergstrom R, et al: Little League survey: The Eugene study. *Am J Sports Med* 1976;4:201-209.
5. Gugenheim JJ, Stanley RF, Woods GW, et al: Little League survey: The Houston study. *Am J Sports Med* 1976;4:189-199.
6. Zarcznyj B, Shattuck LJM, Mast TA, et al: *Am J Sports Med* 1980;8:318-324.
7. Grana WA: Summary of 1978–1979 injury registry for Oklahoma secondary schools. *OSMA J* 1979;72:369-372.
8. Curtin J, Neville RMK: Hand injuries due to soccer. *The Hand* 1976;8:93-95.
9. Delman BJ, et al: Boxing injuries in the army. *J of the Royal Army Medical Corps* 1981;129:32-37.
10. Shields CL, Zomar VD: Analysis of professional football injuries. *Contemp Orthop* 1982;4:90-95.
11. Bogumill GP: A morphologic study of the relationship of collateral ligaments to growth plates in the digits. *J Hand Surg* 1983;8:74-79.
12. Campbell CS: Gamekeeper's thumb. *J Bone Joint Surg* 1955;37:148-149.
13. Stener B: Skeletal injuries associated with rupture of the ulnar collateral ligament of the metacarpophalangeal joint of the thumb. *Acta Chir Scand* 1963;125:583-586.
14. Stener B: Displacement of the ruptured ulnar collateral ligament of the metacarpophalangeal joint of the thumb. *J Bone Joint Surg* 1962; 44B:869-879.
15. McCue FC, Honner R, Johnson MC, et al: Athletic injuries of the proximal interphalangeal joint requiring surgical treatment. *J Bone Joint Surg (Am)* 1970;52:937-956.
16. Mosher J: Flexor and extensor tendon injuries in Pettrone FA (ed). American Academy of Orthopaedic Surgeons *Symposium on Upper Extremity Injuries in Athletes*. St. Louis, CV Mosby, 1984, pp 114-121.
17. Leddy J, Packer J: Avulsion of the profundus tendon insertion in athletes. *J Hand Surg* 1977;2:66-69.
18. Leddy J: Avulsions of the flexor digitorum profundus. *Hand Clin* 1985;1:77-83.
19. Robins PR, Dobyns JH: Avulsion of the insertion of the flexor digitorum profundus tendon associated with fracture of the distal phalanx: American Academy of Orthopaedic Surgeons *Symposium on Tendon Surgery of the Hand*. St. Louis, CV Mosby, 1975.
20. Smith JH Jr: Avulsion of a profundus tendon with simultaneous intraarticular fracture of the distal phalanx: Case report. *J Hand Surg* 1981;6:600-601.
21. Honner R: The late management of the isolated lesion of the flexor digitorum profundus tendon. *The Hand* 1975;7:171-174.
22. Eckhardt WA, Palmer AK: Recurrent dislocation of extensor carpi ulnaris tendon. *J Hand Surg* 1981;6:629-631.
23. Hastings H, Simmons BP: Hand fractures in children. *Clin Orthop* 1984;188:120-130.
24. Salter RB, Harris R: Injuries involving the epiphyseal plate. *J Bone Joint Surg* 1963;45A:587-622.
25. Stuart HC, Pyle SI, Cornoni J, et al: *Pediatrics* 1962;237-249.
26. Simmons BP, Lovallo JL: Hand and wrist injuries in children. *Clin Sports Med* 1988;7:495-512.
27. Light TR: Injury to the immature carpus. *Hand Clin* 1988;4:415-424.
28. Vahvanen V, Westerlund M: Fracture of the carpal scaphoid in children. *Acta Orthop Scand* 1980;51:909-913.
29. Christodoulou AG, Colton CL: Scaphoid fractures in children. *J Ped Orthop* 1986;6:37-39.
30. Pick RY, Segal D: Carpal scaphoid fracture and nonunion in an eight-year-old child. *J Bone Joint Surg* 1983;65:1188-1189.

31. Southcott R, Rosman MA: Nonunion of carpal scaphoid fractures in children. *J Bone Joint Surg* 1977;59:20-23.

32. Stewart MJ: Fractures of the carpal navicular (scaphoid). *J Bone Joint Surg* 1954;36:998-1006.

33. McCoy GF, Graham HK, Piggot J: Nonunion of fractures of the carpal scaphoid in a child. *Ulster Med J* 1956;56:66-68.

34. Louis DS, Calhoun TP, Garn SM, et al: Congenital bipartite scaphoid–fact or fiction? *J Bone Joint Surg* 1976;58:1008-1112.

35. Anderson WJ: Simultaneous fracture of the scaphoid and capitate in a child. *J Hand Surg* 1987;12:271-273.

36. Gouldesbrough C: A case of fracture of scaphoid and os magnum in a boy ten years old. *Lancet* 1916;2:792.

37. Young TB: Isolated fracture of the capitate in a 10-year-old boy. *Injury* 1986;17:133-134.

38. Larson B, Light T, Ogden J: Nonunion and ischemic necrosis of the ossifying carpus. *J Hand Surg* 1987;12:122-127.

39. Gerard FM: Post-traumatic carpal instability in a young child. *J Bone Joint Surg* 1980;62:131-133.

40. Peiro A, Martos F, Mut T, et al: Trans-scaphoid perilunate dislocation in a child. *Acta Orthop Scand* 1981;52:31-34.

Chapter 20

Injuries to the Hip and Pelvis

Lyle J. Micheli, MD

Injuries to the hip and pelvis are relatively common in the young athlete.[1,2] They are often quite different in pattern from those seen in adult athletes. Thus, the special diagnostic and therapeutic implications of such injuries in the young athlete require special attention from physicians.[3,4]

As in the adult, these injuries can be the result of two quite different mechanisms, single-impact macrotrauma or repetitive microtrauma (the so-called overuse injury).[4,5] Occasionally, a combination of these two mechanisms may contribute to injury in the young athlete. For example, a child with a low-grade ache over the rim of the ilium may experience a sudden acute exacerbation of pain, at exactly the same site, with associated swelling and obvious acute tissue injury, after landing a triple jump in a figure-skating competition.

These injuries can be conveniently divided into pelvic and hip joint injuries, with subdivisions of macrotrauma and overuse injuries.

Pelvic Injuries

Macrotrauma Acute macrotrauma to the pelvic region most commonly involves the overlying soft tissue and musculotendinous attachments of the pelvis. Contusions to the subcutaneous tissue or muscle aponeurosis are common and painful. A contusion over the iliac rim ("hip pointer") can be painful enough to require the young athlete to abstain from participation in contact sports such as football or to use special protection over the area of injury to prevent further exacerbation of the injury.[6,7] Development of a frank, necrotizing centrum of these areas of contusions is rare in this age group, and aspiration or evacuation is rarely, if ever, required. Conservative treatment such as icing, relative immobilization, and protection is useful.

Intrinsic, extrinsic, or a combination of intrinsic and extrinsic overload to the muscle-tendon units inserting on the pelvis may occasionally result in an injury in the tendinous substance, as in the hamstrings. In this instance, the diagnosis and rehabilitation of the muscle-tendon strain are similar to those in the older athlete. A much more specific injury encountered in the young athlete, however, is a frank apophyseal avulsion. This may involve the anterosuperior iliac spine where the sartorius inserts, avulsion of the ischial apophysis where the hamstrings insert, the anteroinferior iliac spine where the rectus femoris inserts, or a frank avulsion of the entire iliac crest.[8-11]

The initial diagnosis is often based on the site of pain and tenderness. Radiographic findings are confirmatory.

Nonsurgical management (rest, ice, compression, and elevation) is usually best, followed by slow, progressive restoration of strength and range of motion. This generally results in progressive healing of tissue and restoration of function.[3]

Some investigators believe that a large avulsion of the ischium should be treated with early surgical reduction and fixation but others disagree.[12]

In rare instances, however, this injury may result in persistent pain and functional disability, probably because of fibrous union at the site, particularly if the avulsion is large.[11] In such cases, surgical excision of the painful nonunion may provide progressive restoration of function. Also, if the avulsion of the anterior iliac spine produces subsequent bony healing and overgrowth, significantly limiting abduction and forward flexion, excision of the overlying bony fragment can restore satisfactory function.

Sports-related macrotraumatic fractures or fracture-dislocations of the pelvic ring are rare except in equestrian events.[13-16] In such injuries, of course, management involves determining the relative stability of the fracture and the need for reduction and fixation. Considerations in such sports-related fractures are the same as those in fractures from other causes.

Overuse Injuries   Overuse injuries from repetitive microtrauma about the pelvis appear to be increasing. Apophyseal pain at the site of the iliac crest, or iliac apophysitis, occurs in young skaters and runners.[3,6] Similar pains occur at the insertion of the sartorius on the anterosuperior iliac spine and, occasionally, over the ischium at the insertion of the hamstrings.

In these instances, altering training intensity and restoring the flexibility and the strength of the involved muscle groups have been sufficient to resolve these symptoms, although iliac crest symptoms in particular can be long-lasting.

Another overuse injury, one that is encountered more often in the preadolescent or adolescent athlete, is osteitis pubis.[17] This may be manifested as an adductus strain in the young hockey player or football player. It appears to be particularly associated with running on hard surfaces. The initial diagnosis may be difficult. Occasionally the area over the anterior margin of the symphysis pubis is extremely tender. A radionuclide bone scan can help confirm the diagnosis.

The management of osteitis pubis can be difficult. Occasionally, complete bed rest may be required for a short period, followed by progressive crutch gait training. Anti-inflammatory drugs may be useful. Hydrotherapy and water training are also particularly useful in relieving the stress of this condition until symptoms have subsided.

Stress fractures about the pelvis of the young athlete may also be encountered.[18] Stress fractures of the pubic ramus occur in young runners, particularly female runners; once again, radionuclide scanning can help diagnose such conditions. In the rare cases of sacroiliac strain in young runners, the diagnosis is generally made on the basis of careful physical examination, pattern of injury, and radionuclide scanning.

Hip Injuries

Macrotrauma   Fractures of the femur and femoral neck usually result from severe trauma,[19-22] but they can be sports-related. Several frankly displaced femoral neck fractures have been reported in children who had pre-existing hip pain and, most likely, stress fractures.[23,24]

As with femoral neck fractures of any origin in the child, displaced fractures require proper early reduction and internal fixation to attain union and to protect the vascular supply of the femoral head.[21]

Acute physeal injuries at the hip rarely result from athletic trauma.[20] They most commonly occur in a child with a chronic progressive state, such as a slipped capital femoral epiphysis, after a superimposed episode of trauma during an athletic event.[25,26] The management of these injuries is, of course, similar to that of slipped capital femoral epiphysis of any origin. The superimposed acute trauma may increase the need for partial or complete reduction by means of simple traction or surgery.

Hip dislocations in the young athlete, like hip dislocations caused by macrotrauma in general, are usually posterior and superior. Rarely, an inferior dislocation may be encountered.[27]

The key to satisfactory management of this condition is prompt recognition. The child, who is generally in a position of adduction interrotation and limb shortening, must be transported as quickly as possible to an appropriate facility for careful radiographic assessment of the injury. Once a diagnosis has been made, a careful neurologic examination should be performed to determine the status of the injury and the potential for an associated sciatic nerve injury. Closed reduction with the patient under anesthesia should be performed to lessen the risk of avascular necrosis. If necessary, postoperative computed tomographic scans are obtained to confirm that there is no associated rim fracture or interposition of soft tissues that might prevent symmetric reduction.

Postoperative immobilization is a matter of some debate. Some authors have recommended postoperative, nonweightbearing crutch gait for as long as 12 weeks to lessen the chances of avascular necrosis.[27] The relative risk of avascular necrosis probably depends primarily on the disruption of or transient interference with the blood supply of the capital epiphyses during the period of dislocation and is probably not associated with postoperative management. Most authors recommend four to six weeks of protected crutch gait to allow satisfactory healing of the capsule. Recurrent dislocations are extremely rare in this age group.[27]

Postinjury complications include avascular necrosis and neurologic dysfunction. This condition is a major musculoskeletal disruption in the athletically active child, and vigorous contact-sport competitions should be prohibited for 12 months after the injury.

Another macrotraumatic injury occurring at the hip is avulsion of the lesser trochanter. This can be extremely painful in the young athlete. Like avulsions about the hip and pelvis in general, these occur in particularly tight tissues of young athletes, often during a growth spurt.

Management, again, consists of initial relative rest of the area and slow, progressive restoration of function. Surgical reduction is not required, as healing appears to occur inevitably without residual symptoms of any significance and without loss of function.

Overuse Injuries The young athlete or dancer who has "snapping hip" generally has one of two distinct entities. The more common is iliotibial band friction syndrome, particularly with abduction elevation of the extremity. The young athlete often complains that the hip is "going out of place."[28]

A program of directed stretching exercises, anti-inflammatory drugs, and icing is particularly useful. In rare cases, surgical release of the iliotibial band is required to relieve these symptoms.

The second type of snapping hip occurs more medially. It is often found in ballet dancers who perform *developes* or *ronds de jambe*. Recent studies have suggested that this entity is the result of a snapping of the iliopsoas over the neck of the femur and associated tenosynovitis.[28] Others have raised concern about the possibility of a partial subluxation of the hip and acetabulum or actual labral instability in these instances.

A specific antilordosis therapy program, along with stretching and strengthening of the hip external rotators and the iliopsoas, almost always provides symptomatic relief and rids the hip of the snapping.

Other Conditions

It is imperative that the physician remember that young athletically active individuals are subject to more general afflictions occurring about the hip and pelvis, such as Legg-Calvé-Perthes disease. In athletically active children who develop hip pain secondary to nontraumatic disease, diagnosis is often delayed because the symptoms are attributed to athletic overuse. Similarly, neoplasms about the hip and pelvis must always be ruled out in the athletically active child. Spontaneous development of local sepsis of the pelvic region must be kept in mind as a possible cause of pain in the young athlete. Diskitis may also be confused with pelvic disease. Leukemia and neuroblastoma may be manifested as hip pain. Similarly, a slipped capital femoral epiphysis can appear as knee pain in the athletically active individual.[2]

References

1. Izant RJ Jr, Hubay CA: The annual injury of 15,000,000 children: A limited study of childhood accidental injury and death. *J Trauma* 1966;6:65-74.
2. Waters PM, Millis MB: Hip and pelvic injuries in the young athlete. *Clin Sports Med* 1988;7:513-526.
3. Micheli LJ: Sites of overuse injury, in Lovell WW, Winter RB (eds): *Pediatric Orthopaedics*, ed 2. Philadelphia, JB Lippincott, 1986.
4. Micheli LJ: Overuse injuries in children's sports: The growth factor. *Orthop Clin North Am* 1983;14:337.
5. Adrish JG: Overuse syndromes of the lower extremity in youth sports, in Boileau R (ed): *Advances in Pediatric Sports Sciences*. Champaign, Human Kinetics Publishers.
6. Clancy WG Jr, Foltz AS: Iliac apophysitis and stress fractures in adolescent runners. *Am J Sports Med* 1976;4:214-218.
7. Garrick JG: Sports medicine. *Pediatr Clin North Am* 1986;33:1541-1550.
8. Fernbach SK, Wilkinson RH: Avulsion injuries of pelvis and proximal femur. *AJR* 1981;137:581-584.
9. Godshall RW, Hansen CA: Incomplete avulsion of a portion of the iliac epiphysis: An injury of young athletes. *J Bone Joint Surg* 1973;55A:1301-1302.
10. Metzmaker JN, Pappas AM: Avulsion fractures of the pelvis. *Am J Sports Med* 1985;13:349-358.
11. Schlonsky J, Olix ML: Functional disability following avulsion fracture of the ischial epiphysis: Report of two cases. *J Bone Joint Surg* 1972;54A:641-644.
12. Canale ST, King RE: Pelvic and hip fractures, in Rockwood CA Jr, Wilkins KE, King RE (eds): *Fractures: Vol 3. Fractures in Children*. Philadelphia, JB Lippincott, 1984, pp 733-843.
13. Blatter R: Fractures of the pelvis and acetabulum, in Weber BG, Brunner C, Freuler F (eds): *Treatment of Fractures in Children and Adolescents*. Berlin, Springer-Verlag, 1980.
14. Bryan WJ, Tullos HS: Pediatric pelvic fractures: Review of 52 patients. *J Trauma* 1979;19:799-805.
15. Torode I, Zieg D: Pelvic fractures in children. *J Pediatr Orthop* 1985;5:76-84.
16. Watts HG: Fractures of the pelvis in children. *Orthop Clin North Am* 1976;7:615-624.
17. Koch RA, Jackson DW: Pubic symphysitis in runners: A report of two cases. *Am J Sports Med* 1981;9:62-63.
18. Latshaw RF, Kantner TR, Kalenak A, et al: A pelvic stress fracture in a female jogger: A case report. *Am J Sports Med* 1981;9:54-56.
19. Bortzy A: Fractures of the proximal femur, in Weber BG, Brunner C, Freuler F (eds): *Treatment of Fractures in Children and Adolescents*. Berlin, Springer-Verlag, 1980.
20. Larson RL: Epiphyseal injuries in the adolescent athlete. *Orthop Clin North Am* 1973;4:839-851.
21. Ogden JA: Trauma, hip development, and vascularity, in Tronzo RG (ed): *Surgery of the Hip Joint*, ed 2. New York, Springer-Verlag, 1984, vol 1, pp 145-180.
22. Tronzo RG: Fractures in children, in Tronzo RG (ed): *Surgery of the Hip Joint*, ed 2. New York, Springer-Verlag, 1984, vol 1, pp 191-202.
23. Devas MB: Stress fractures of the femoral neck. *J Bone Joint Surg* 1965;47B:728-738.

24. Hajek MR, Noble HB: Stress fractures of the femoral neck in joggers: Case report and review of the literature. *Am J Sports Med* 1982;10:112-116.

25. Weinstein SL, Morrissy RT, Crawford AH: Slipped capital femoral epiphysis, in Murray JA (ed): American Academy of Orthopaedic Surgeons *Instructional Course Lectures, XXXIII.* St. Louis, CV Mosby, 1984, pp 310-349.

26. Wenger DR: Slipped capital femoral epiphysis, in Tronzo RG (ed): *Surgery of the Hip Joint,* ed 2. New York, Spinger-Verlag, 1984, vol 1, pp 247-272.

27. Offierski CM: Traumatic dislocations of the hip in children. *J Bone Joint Surg* 1981;63B:194-197.

28. Micheli LJ: Dance injuries: The back, hip and pelvis, in Clarkson PM, Skrinar M (eds): *The Science of Dance Training.* Champaign, Human Kinetics Publishers, 1988.

Chapter 21

Injuries to the Knee

William A. Grana, MD

Knee disorders in skeletally immature athletes present unique problems in diagnosis and treatment. Although lower-extremity injuries occur less often in children than in older athletes,[1] about 10% to 15% of all lower-extremity injuries occur in athletes 14 years of age and younger. These injuries are most common in cutting sports such as soccer, football, and basketball.[2]

Diagnostic Information

No information is yet available on the use of arthrograms, computed tomographic scans, bone scans, magnetic resonance imaging, or ultrasound as diagnostic tools specific to children's injuries. Each of these tests will undoubtedly have some value in diagnosing particular problems and ensuring accurate diagnoses. However, at present the best diagnostic information that can be obtained comes from the patient history, the physical examination, and the use of arthroscopy.

Arthroscopy is of particular value in diagnosing hemarthrosis. The use of arthroscopy obviates the need for arthrotomy and increases diagnostic accuracy in children even more than in adults.[3,4] Arthroscopy in the child's knee frequently reveals no surgically treatable problem and often disproves the clinical diagnosis. Specifically, arthroscopy is valuable for localizing the lesion in both the anatomic structure and the compartment involved and for exactly defining the lesion. It also demonstrates that there is a credible lesion present and that the patient's problem is not a functional one.[5]

Meniscal Injury and Repair

Meniscal injury is rare in the skeletally immature patient but becomes more common as adolescence proceeds.[6] Arthroscopy and arthrography can confirm the diagnosis of meniscal tear.[7]

The child's meniscus differs from the adult's in its vascularity and cellularity. Vessels are most prominent in the peripheral third but are

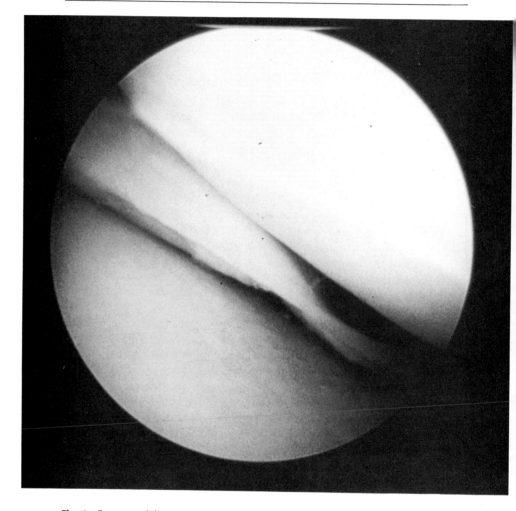

Fig. 1. *Because of the unique anatomic characteristics of the meniscus, every effort should be made to repair meniscal injury in children in order to maintain the structure and function of the meniscus.*

present throughout the meniscus. Because of this unique anatomic characteristic, every effort should be made to repair meniscal injury in children and to maintain the structure and function of the meniscus (Fig. 1).

Results of meniscectomy show it is not a benign procedure in a child. In a study of 59 knees in 49 patients with an average age of 13 years and with an average follow-up of 7½ years, only 42% were asymptomatic and only 27% were free of Fairbanks' radiographic changes.[8] Again, every effort should be made to preserve the meniscus.

Meniscal healing depends on the type of tear and the age of the patient. Of peripheral-third tears, 80% to 90% heal successfully. Preservation of the meniscus is particularly important in the unstable knee to protect the joint surface and to return stability. Surgical complications from meniscal repair in children are similar to those seen in adults, including neurovascular injury in the lateral compartment and injury to the saphenous nerve and vein on the medial side. Injury can be avoided by staying anterior to the biceps, with the femur on the lateral side and the pes anserinus on the medial side. Entrapment of the saphenous nerve is the most common complication seen.[9-11]

Discoid Meniscus

Discoid lateral meniscus was first described by Young[12] in 1889. In 1910, Kroiss[13] described the "snapping knee" syndrome. The origin of discoid meniscus is controversial. Smillie[14] described it as the persistence of a disk-shaped meniscus that is present at birth. However, Kaplan's[15] explanation is accepted by most: the discoid meniscus is a normal meniscus with abnormal attachments to the periphery of the joint.

Two types of discoid menisci are described depending on their posterior attachment. One type is peripherally attached to the capsule; the other's only attachment is through Wrisberg's ligament. It is the latter type that produces the snapping syndrome.

The discoid meniscus is not only abnormally shaped, but also hypertrophic and thickened. Where the peripheral attachment is complete, size may vary as well. Completely attached discoid menisci are asymptomatic but may have sustained radial-type tears requiring saucerization as treatment. Treatment for the Wrisberg's ligament type with "snapping syndrome" is complete meniscectomy.[12,13,16] Partial resection of a discoid meniscus to more normal meniscal contours will result in a smooth rim as adaptive changes occur. However, further meniscal tears may occur just as in the normally shaped meniscus.[17]

Medial-Shelf Syndrome

Medial-shelf syndrome, or symptomatic plica, can occur in the young patient. About half of the cases diagnosed are sports-related.[18] Mital and Hayden[19] noted 15 patients between 11 and 16 years of age with medial-shelf syndrome that was relieved by surgical excision. This syndrome is a less common cause of internal derangement problems in the child's knee than in that of the adolescent. Medial-shelf syndrome may be mistaken for a meniscal tear or a patellofemoral problem such as a tracking abnormality. The treatment of choice is complete excision; mild symptoms recur in 30% of patients.[20]

Patellofemoral Problems

Although patellofemoral pain problems are common in adolescents through middle-aged patients, they are rare in the child. Patellar dis-

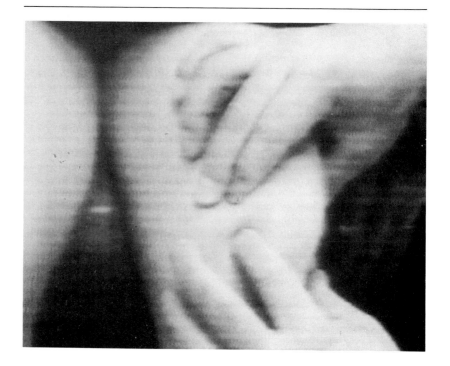

Fig. 2. *Instability or tracking problems, which are seen in the older child and adolescent, are rarely seen in the school-age child with patellofemoral pain syndrome.*

location may occur in a child but most often results from athletic trauma suffered later in life. In a prospective study, fewer than 10% of patients with patellofemoral pain were under 13 years of age, and all of these patients were treated nonsurgically.[21]

Patellofemoral pain in children is often self-limited because the child will restrict activity to avoid the pain. The pain is commonly caused by relative quadriceps dysplasia, which results in malalignment and lateral tracking. This condition can be treated with almost universally good results by an extension exercise routine and rest. The problem is distinct from the more common patellar tracking disorders—instability, patellar compression, and chondromalacia—seen in older patients (Fig. 2).[22]

Several other extensor mechanism problems that occur in the child require mention here. These problems can be thought of as overuse problems resulting from microtrauma. Osgood-Schlatter disease is an avulsion injury of the tibial apophysis or a traction of apophysitis with heterotopic bone formation as a result of microfractures of the tibial tubercle. The specific cause is unknown. The majority of patients respond to nonsurgical treatment management: restriction of activity, immobilization, nonsteroidal anti-inflammatory agents, and exercises to improve quadriceps strength and power.[23] In those patients who do not respond to these treatments (10% to 15%), loose fragments are surgically excised with little or no risk of growth-center injury.[24] Sinding-Larsen-Johansson syndrome is a variant of this same problem that occurs at the proximal end of the patella. Again, the treatment is primarily nonsurgical.

Patellar sleeve fracture is an avulsion of a fracture, usually as the result of forceful extension. The physical examination usually reveals a high-riding patella unable to extend actively. The fracture also occurs through the bone with a sleeve of cartilage. For the displaced fragment, open repair is necessary to avoid an extensor lag.[25]

Osteochondritis Dissecans

Osteochondritis dissecans of the patella usually occurs in persons more than 16 years old but can occur in those 13 years of age or younger. In the fragmented or loose lesion, curettement is the treatment of choice. If the articular surface is intact, drilling of the subchondral bone is the preferred treatment. In either instance the results are guarded.[26]

Most cases of osteochondritis dissecans (75%) occur in the knees of young male athletes. Paré described loose bodies in the knee in 1558 and Pagent described the quiet necrosis associated with these loose bodies in 1870. Konig described the pathology of osteochondritis dissecans and its occurrence as a result of trauma in 1888.[27]

Nonetheless, the etiology of this condition has remained controversial, with trauma, ischemia, aberrant ossification centers, or epiphyseal abnormalities of genetic origin all being considered as causes. None has been shown to be an exclusive cause; most practitioners accept that some degree of trauma, along with constitutional predisposition, is necessary for osteochondritis dissecans to occur.

"Wilson's sign" in the physical examination is believed to be pathognomonic, and on plain radiographs the lateral and tunnel views are believed to be of greatest value. Arthrograms may show separation of the fragment in the interface between the fragment and the defect, while a bone scan may show late-phase intensity caused by loosening and focal hyperemia.[28] Uptake in the bone scan is proportional to the severity of loosening. Computerized blood flow analysis can be done with a bone scan to provide prognostic information about healing. Increased flow indicates healing while decreased blood flow indicates a poor prognosis.[29] Magnetic resonance imaging has been of questionable value in these lesions because it is difficult to distinguish the fluid at the interface of the fragment in the bed or separation of the fragment from the bed.

Treatment depends on the age of the patient. In a skeletally mature patient, surgical treatment is more often indicated.[27] In the child, nonsurgical treatment is the rule, with rest, restriction of activity, and radiographic follow-up of the course of the lesion. Stable fragments may be drilled or fixed; loose bodies should be removed. Newer techniques with the use of Herbert screws and other specialized devices may provide better compression and promote healing[30] (Fig. 3).

Ligament Injury

Ligament injuries account for less than 1% of knee injuries in studies of the skeletally immature patient. Ligament injuries are distinguished from physeal injuries through stress radiographs.[31] These injuries do not usually occur as a result of sports trauma. They are often part of multisystem problems and are frequently overlooked. Associated injuries include intercondylar fracture, tibial tubercle avulsion, and anterior cruciate ligament rupture. Surgical repair of the complete lesion with meniscal preservation is recommended. Some degree of laxity usually occurs after ligament repair.[32]

Both anterior cruciate ligament tears and collateral ligament injuries can occur in the skeletally immature patient. Intra-articular reconstruction is the preferred treatment, although concerns about the physes have led some surgeons to use an over-the-top technique or extra-articular reconstruction. The clinician must be aware of congenital absence of the anterior cruciate ligament. Arthroscopy can rule out this absence as well as intercondylar eminence fracture. Again, some degree of instability following repair or reconstruction of the ligament is the rule.[32-34]

Fractures

Femoral Physeal Injury   Distal femoral physeal injury is associated with a much higher incidence of growth discrepancy than injuries in other anatomic areas. Therefore, Salter I and II fractures are not benign in this area and must be viewed with suspicion. Complications can include vascular disturbance, limitation of motion, and instability.[35]

The mechanism of injury is hyperextension and torsion. The proximal fragment is usually displaced medially. Sports trauma is a frequent cause of injury, particularly from jumping sports such as the high jump, hurdling, or basketball.[35]

The general prognosis of these fractures corresponds to the Salter-Harris classification: groups I and II injuries have a better prognosis than groups III, IV, and V. However, any physeal injury in the femoral area carries a poorer prognosis than one in another area of the body.[36,37]

Limb-length discrepancy is not uncommon after fractures of this type even though the average age at the time of this injury is 11 to 12 years. A leg-length discrepancy of 1 cm or more occurs in 40% to 60% of patients with physeal injury when the fracture is displaced more than half the diameter of the bone and is not reduced. Anatomic reduction eliminates the problem in almost all cases.[33,35]

Another common problem is angular deformity. About one-third of patients show more than 5 degrees of varus valgus alignment. However, the deformity is not usually severe enough to require surgical

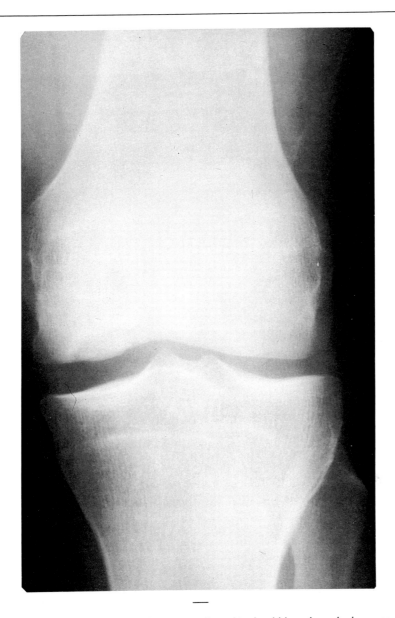

Fig. 3. *A stable osteochondral fragment such as this should be salvaged whenever possible. Drilling or fixation of the fragment is the best approach to maintain the articular surface.*

intervention. Loss of motion is usually not incapacitating following physeal injury; laxity occurs in 25% to 35% of patients.[33,35]

Tibial Physeal Injury Proximal tibial physeal injury accounts for only 0.5% of all physeal injuries. Stabilization by the collateral ligaments

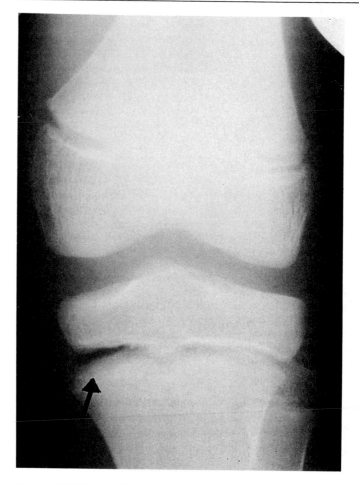

Fig. 4. *Proximal tibial physeal injury is rare but can occur and is a cause of collateral ligament laxity, particularly on the medial side. Stress radiographs are mandatory to evaluate these injuries.*

contributes to this low occurrence (Fig. 4). The patellar tendon is involved in avulsion injury of the proximal tibial apophysis as discussed below. Patients with proximal tibial physeal injury are typically 12 to 14 years old.[38] Stress radiographs are used to diagnose the problem. Complications are similar to those of distal femoral physeal injury. However, intra-articular and arterial injuries are more common in these fractures. An angiogram should be considered in making the diagnosis.[36,37]

Tibial Tubercle Avulsion   Tibial tubercle avulsion injury occurs because maturation makes distinct changes in the fibrocartilage of the tibial apophysis. This cartilage becomes columnar in nature and weak in tensile loading. Injury commonly occurs to those 12 to 16 years of age.

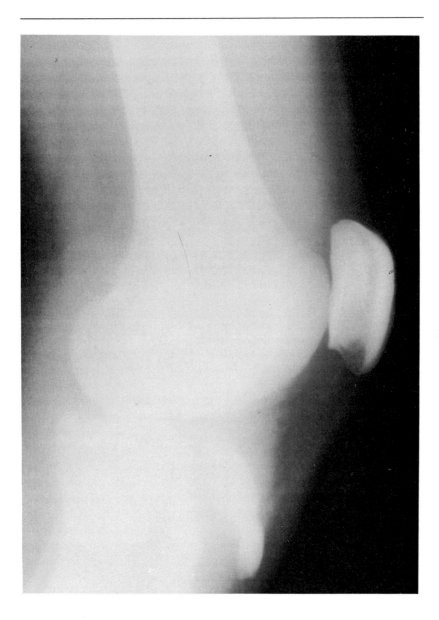

Fig. 5. *Tibial tubercle avulsion which involves the surface of the joint must be treated by open reduction/internal fixation to re-establish the articular surface.*

Forceful contraction of the quadriceps, such as coming down from a jump with the knee flexed, often results in an injury of this type. Open reduction of any displacement is the treatment of choice. Follow-up of undisplaced fractures is important to disclose displaced fragments. Premature closure of the apophysis is uncommon. The prime concern of

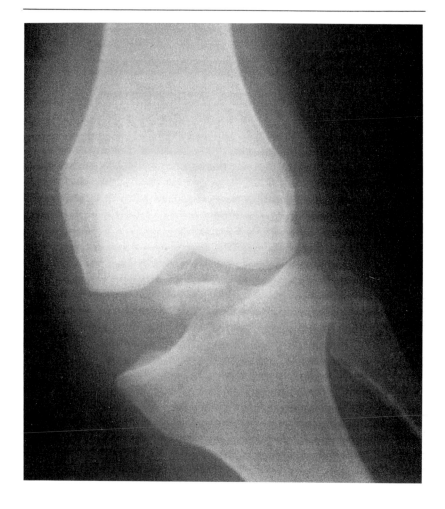

Fig. 6. *Intercondylar eminence fracture is a cause of anterior laxity in the adolescent and child. Displaced fragments must be treated by open reduction/internal fixation. When ligamentous injuries occur in the pediatric patient, intercondylar eminence fracture is also common.*

treatment should be to re-establish any articular surface abnormality (Fig. 5).[39]

Intercondylar Eminence Fracture   Intercondylar eminence fracture is usually seen in children under 15 years of age; 30% of these injuries occur in some kind of fall (Fig. 6). Clinically, patients characteristically have hemarthrosis and decreased ability to bear weight on the injured limb.[40] One-third of patients will have symptoms of giving way and two-thirds of these will have decreased their activities because of anterior cruciate ligament instability. Nonunion of the displaced fracture is common. Salter II and III fractures usually require surgery to prevent bad unions and correct instabilities. However, open reduction and internal fixation of the displaced fragment may not relieve all symptoms if laxity results from plastic deformation of a ligament. In one study, eight of 15 patients had pain and two of 15 had symptoms of subluxation after surgery.[40]

Popliteal Cysts It is important to remember that most popliteal cysts will disappear without surgery and that those removed may recur. In a study of 120 cysts[41], 50 underwent surgery and, of these, 21 recurred. Seventy were treated nonsurgically and 51 caused no problems in 18 months of follow-up.

The causes of popliteal cyst are mechanical and synovial. Juvenile rheumatoid arthritis may be manifest as a popliteal cyst and effusion. Rupture of the cyst may occur, producing severe pain in the calf, indicating an early manifestation of rheumatoid arthritis.[41,42]

Misdiagnoses

Hip problems, infection (particularly gonococcal infection), and synovial problems all must be ruled out in the problem patient with knee pain. Tumors may also occur about the knee. In a review of 36 patients, a tumor was the cause of symptoms in all cases first thought to result from sports trauma.[43] When a patient does not respond to conservative treatment, further evaluation is necessary through the use of bone scans, computed tomographic scans, and magnetic resonance imaging.[43] The most frequent misdiagnoses in patients with knee pain of undetermined cause are chondromalacia and traumatic effusion.[44]

References

1. Kannus P, Jarvinen M: Role of sports in etiology and prognosis of surgically treated acute knee ligament injuries. *Int J Sports Med* 1986;7:39-43.
2. Sandelin J: Acute sports injuries requiring hospital care. *Br J Sports Med* 1986;20:99-102.
3. Eiskjaer S, Larsen ST: Arthroscopy of the knee in children. *Acta Orthop Scand* 1987;58:273-276.
4. Morrissy RT, Eubanks RG, Park JP, et al: Arthroscopy of the knee in children. *Clin Orthop* 1982;162:103-107.
5. Eilert RE: Arthroscopy of the knee joint in children. *Orthop Rev* 1976;5:61-65.
6. Clark CR, Ogden JA: Development of the menisci of the human knee joint: Morphological changes and their potential role in childhood meniscal injury. *J Bone Joint Surg* 1983;65A:538-547.
7. Ritchie DM: Meniscectomy in children. *Aust NZ J Surg* 1966;35:239-241.
8. Zaman M, Leonard MA: Meniscectomy in children: A study of fifty nine knees. *J Bone Joint Surg* 1978;60B:436-437.
9. Barber FA: Meniscus repair: Results of an arthroscopic technique. *Arthroscopy* 1987;3:25-30.
10. DeHaven KE: Meniscus repair: Open vs arthroscopic. *Arthroscopy* 1985;1:173-174.

11. Lynch MA, Henning CE, Glick KR Jr: Knee joint surface changes: Long-term follow-up meniscus tear treatment in stable anterior cruciate ligament reconstructions. *Clin Orthop* 1983;172:148-153.

12. Young RB: The external semilunar cartilage as a complete disc. *Anatomy*, 1889, 179.

13. Kroiss F: Die Verletzungen der Kniegelenkszwischenknorpel und ihrer Verbindungen. *Beitr Klin Chir* 1910;66:598-801.

14. Smillie IS: The congenital discoid meniscus. *J Bone Joint Surg* 1948;30B:671-682.

15. Kaplan EB: Discoid lateral meniscus of the knee joint: Nature, mechanism, and operative treatment. *J Bone Joint Surg* 1957;39A:77-87.

16. Dickhaut SC, DeLee JC: The discoid lateral-meniscus syndrome. *J Bone Joint Surg* 1982;64A:1068-1073.

17. Fujikawa K, Iseki F, Mikura Y: Partial resection of the discoid meniscus in the child's knee. *J Bone Joint Surg* 1981;63B:391-395.

18. Broom MJ, Fulkerson JP: The plica syndrome: A new perspective. *Orthop Clin North Am* 1986;17:279-281.

19. Mital MA, Hayden J: Pain in the knee in children: The medial plica shelf syndrome. *Orthop Clin North Am* 1979;10:713-722.

20. Muse GL, Grana WA, Hollingsworth S: Arthroscopic treatment of medial shelf syndrome. *Arthroscopy* 1985;1:63-67.

21. Yates C, Grana WA: Patellofemoral pain: A prospective study. *Orthopedics* 1986;9:663-667.

22. Grana WA, Kriegshauser LA: Scientific basis of extensor mechanism disorders. *Clin Sports Med* 1985;4:247-257.

23. Mital MA, Matza RA, Cohen J: The so-called unresolved Osgood-Schlatter lesion: A concept based on fifteen surgically treated lesions. *J Bone Joint Surg* 1980;62A:732-739.

24. Griffin PP: The lower limb, in Lovell WW, Winter RB (eds): *Pediatric Orthopaedics*. Philadelphia, JB Lippincott, 1978, vol 2. pp 881-909.

25. Houghton GR, Ackroyd CE: Sleeve fractures of the patella in children: A report of three cases. *J Bone Joint Surg* 1979;61B:165-168.

26. Desai SS, Patel MR, Michelli LJ, et al: Osteochondritis dissecans of the patella. *J Bone Joint Surg* 1987;69B:320-325.

27. Clanton TO, DeLee JC: Osteochondritis dissecans: History, pathophysiology and current treatment concepts. *Clin Orthop* 1982;167:50-64.

28. Mesgarzadeh M, Sapega AA, Bonakdarpour A, et al: Osteochondritis dissecans: Analysis of mechanical stability with radiography, scintigraphy, and MR imaging. *Radiology* 1987;165:775-780.

29. Litchman HM, McCullough RW, Gandsman EJ, et al: Computerized blood flow analysis for decision making in the treatment of osteochondritis dissecans. *J Pediatr Orthop* 1988;8:208-212.

30. Thomson NL: Osteochondritis dissecans and osteochondral fragments managed by Herbert compression screw fixation. *Clin Orthop* 1987;224:71-78.

31. Clanton TO, DeLee JC, Sanders B, et al: Knee ligament injuries in children. *J Bone Joint Surg* 1979;61A:1195-1201.

32. DeLee JC, Curtis R: Anterior cruciate ligament insufficiency in children. *Clin Orthop* 1983;172:112-118.

33. Lipscomb AB, Anderson AF: Tears of the anterior cruciate ligament in adolescents. *J Bone Joint Surg* 1986;68A:19-28.

34. McCarroll JR, Rettig AC, Shelbourne KD: Anterior cruciate ligament injuries in the young athlete with open physes. *Am J Sports Med* 1988;16:44-47.

35. Stephens DC, Louis E, Louis DS: Traumatic separation of the distal femoral epiphyseal cartilage plate. *J Bone Joint Surg* 1974;56A:1383-1390.

36. Lombardo SJ, Harvey JP Jr: Fractures of the distal femoral epiphyses: Factors influencing prognosis. A review of thirty-four cases. *J Bone Joint Surg* 1977;59A:742-751.

37. Shelton WR, Canale ST: Fractures of the tibia through the proximal tibial epiphyseal cartilage. *J Bone Joint Surg* 1979;61A:167-173.

38. Burkhart SS, Peterson HA: Fractures of the proximal tibial epiphysis. *J Bone Joint Surg* 1979;61A:996-1002.

39. Ogden JA, Tross RB, Murphy MJ: Fractures of the tibial tuberosity in adolescents. *J Bone Joint Surg* 1980;62A:205-215.

40. Smith JB: Knee instability after fractures of the intercondylar eminence of the tibia. *J Pediatr Orthop* 1984;4:462-464.

41. Dinham JM: Popliteal cysts in children: The case against surgery. *J Bone Joint Surg* 1975;57B:69-71.

42. Soslow AR: Popliteal cysts in a pediatric patient. *Ann Emerg Med* 1987;16:588-591.

43. Lewis MM, Reilly JF: Sports tumors. *Am J Sports Med* 1987;15:362-365.

44. Ehrlich MG, Zaleske DJ: Pediatric orthopedic pain of unknown origin. *J Pediatr Orthop* 1986;6:460-468.

Chapter 22

Injuries to the Leg, Ankle and Foot

Letha Y. Hunter-Griffin, MD, PhD

General Considerations

Injuries to the leg, ankle, and foot are common in the pediatric athlete. In Garrick and Requa's[1] study of pediatric skiers, two-thirds of the fractures that occurred were in the leg and ankle region. In 1979, Trott[2] reported that foot and ankle injuries accounted for 12.1% of all injuries in an adolescent population in Boston.

Not only do the patterns of injury sustained by children differ from those in adults, but the numbers and types of injuries sustained by young children are different from those seen in adolescents. Adolescents tend to sustain more injuries and more severe injuries than do children. Greater body mass and greater strength have been reported to be major factors in these statistics.

Fractures in the adolescent tend to occur at the physeal area rather than at the diaphyseal area, as in the preadolescent. Rapidly growing adolescent apophyses (heel, knee, the base of the fifth metatarsal) may become inflamed and painful, conditions not found in early childhood.

Acute Injuries

Fractures and Dislocations　Acute bone injuries consist primarily of fractures and dislocations, but the locations and the complications of fractures differ among children, adolescents, and adults.

Tibia　A proximal metaphyseal tibial fracture with intact fibula is common in children. This fracture appears benign, but can develop valgus angulation even if it is appropriately treated. Parents should be aware that the tibia can, through overgrowth of the medial cortex, develop a valgus angulation that may need surgical correction at a later date.

Overgrowth problems of the tibia resulting in limb-length discrepancy are not as common as those in the femur. In younger children with diaphyseal rather than epiphyseal injuries, both lower extremities should

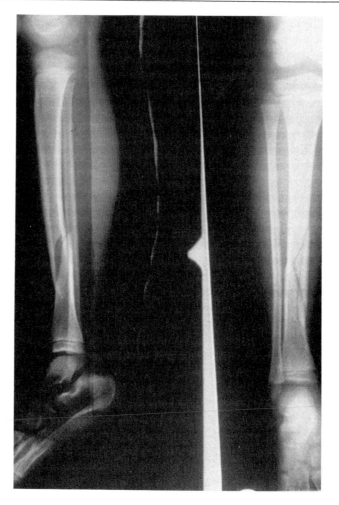

Fig. 1 *Spiral diaphyseal fractures of the femur or tibia in children can lead to leg-length discrepancies from overgrowth.*

be measured after the fracture has healed to identify overgrowth if it does occur.

Figure 1 shows an example of such a fracture. In children, this spiral diaphyseal fracture can usually be treated by closed reduction. Care must be taken to avoid malrotation. Also, after reduction of a tibial/fibular fracture in a child, angular deformities of more than 10 degrees are not acceptable because they can lead to permanent deformity.[3]

Although rotational forces at the ankle generally cause ligamentous injuries in adults, these same forces produce physeal injuries in children. For example, supination plantarflexion injuries can result in physeal injuries to the distal tibia (Fig. 2). Swelling about the physis may be

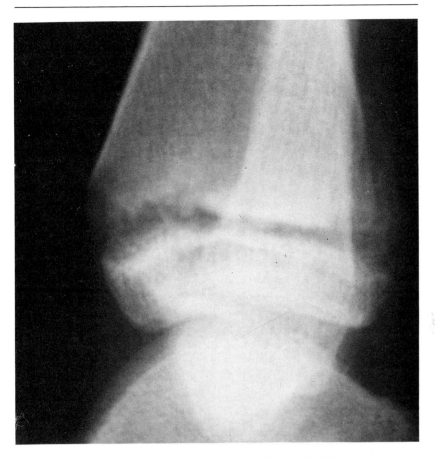

Fig. 2 *Salter I and II fractures of the distal tibia may be initially difficult to see on routine radiographs.*

minimal, but a fracture should always be suspected when a child has had a rotational injury, complains of pain, and has marked tenderness to palpation around the distal tibia. In such cases, the leg should be protected in a short cast as if a fracture had occurred and re-examined radiographically in two weeks. As Gregg and Das[4] stated, "the words 'no fracture seen' in a radiologist's reports do not mean that an epiphyseal separation did not occur."

A Salter II fracture of the distal tibia is usually amenable to closed reduction and does not result in growth abnormalities. Gentle closed manipulation, which may require general anesthesia, is recommended. After reduction, a long leg cast is applied and weightbearing is prohibited for several weeks. Total healing time is generally six weeks.

Salter III and IV fractures of the distal tibia may be associated with premature closure of the physis, even as long as 18 to 24 months after injury (Fig. 3). These children must be monitored for several years be-

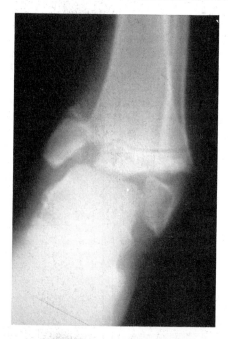

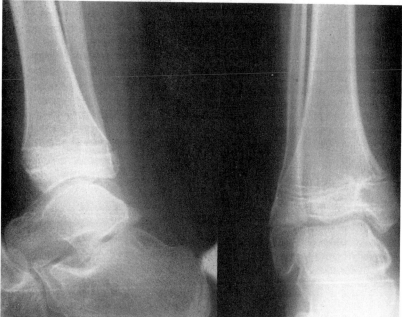

Fig. 3 *Salter IV displaced fracture (top) in a 9-year-old child resulted in early asymmetric closure of the physeal plate (bottom).*

cause of the possibilities of irregular closure of the physeal plate, which may result in limb malalignment, and of premature closure of the entire physis, which may result in a limb-length discrepancy.

Anatomic reduction of types III and IV physeal injuries to the distal tibia is needed to prevent bony bridging across the physis, leading to premature closure. However, parents should be warned that even if an anatomic reduction is accomplished, premature closure may still result because of damage to the growing cells at the time of injury.[5] Growth arrest secondary to a physeal injury may not be totally preventable, but it should be recognized and treated appropriately when it occurs.

As the medial aspect of the distal tibial physis closes at the end of adolescence, external rotational injuries may result in a fracture of the anterolateral quadrant of the tibial physis, a Salter III injury. This fracture can be reduced by internally rotating the foot; if displacement is still greater than 2 mm, however, surgical intervention with reduction and smooth pinning is recommended.

Fibula   Salter I and II fractures of the distal fibula are the most common fractures in children. They result from supination-inversion injuries. There may be minimal swelling. If swelling is present, it is usually localized over the tip of the fibula instead of anterior or inferior to the fibula as it is in ligament injuries. Similarly, the pain is localized to the tip of the fibula, rather than diffusely about the area anteroinferior to it. Minimal widening of the physis may be the only radiographic sign, and it may be subtle.

Suspected Salter I or II injuries to the distal fibula should be protected by short leg casts for several weeks, and then re-evaluated. The duration of nonweightbearing immobilization in fibular physeal injuries has not been definitively established. Generally, only partial weightbearing is permitted for several weeks, with a total healing time of approximately six weeks for this injury.

Fractures of the metatarsals and phalanges in children occur during sports participation. They typically occur when one child jumps on another child's foot. Surgical correction is rarely needed. These fractures may be difficult to recognize, as there are multiple growth centers in the foot. Comparison views of the other foot may be helpful. Also, a careful physical examination usually elicits the localized area of tenderness, targeting the area of the radiograph to be studied more closely.

Protective devices or orthoses that allow an early return to sports after injuries to the foot are seldom designed for children. Children's foot fractures heal rapidly (three to four weeks) and it is frequently best to wait until the fracture is completely healed before permitting the child to return to sports.

Jones fractures, or stress fractures through the proximal third of the fifth metatarsals, are rare in children and young teenagers. This fracture does occur in the older teenager (Fig. 4). It is associated with a high rate of nonunion. Recommended treatment is six weeks in a nonweightbearing cast, followed by six weeks in a weightbearing cast or protective orthosis. Use of the orthosis can be continued as the athlete progresses into walking and running activities. Because of the high rate of nonunion

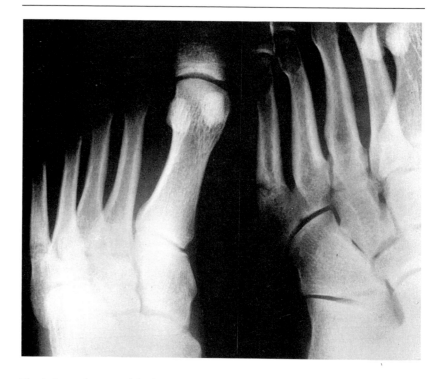

Fig. 4 *Stress fracture of the base of the fifth metatarsal, a Jones fracture.*

in these fractures, some surgeons recommend immediate open reduction with internal fixation and bone graft, particularly if the fracture has a sclerotic margin when initially diagnosed. In the absence of these early radiographic findings, however, conservative care is recommended.

Soft-Tissue Injuries

The most common acute soft-tissue injuries in children are contusions. Blisters and lacerations are also common and deserve special attention in children. Growing children require properly fitting shoes. Shoes can be outgrown rapidly, sometimes within a season. Parents may buy shoes too large for a child so that the child can "grow into them." Blisters can result if shoes are either too tight or too loose.

Physicians and parents should periodically examine children's feet for blisters, and make certain that proper care is instituted. If the child is older, the parents should stress to the child the need for proper shoes and teach the child how to care for a blistered area. Clean socks should always be worn.

Second skin, moleskin, and antiskid pads may help protect children who develop blisters frequently despite proper shoes. Because trainers are usually not available and coaches may not be aware of foot problems, the physician who performs the preseason screening physical examination should advise parents about first-aid measures to prevent and treat common foot problems.

Athlete's foot should be treated aggressively with an antifungal agent as it is contagious and may spread among those who share a locker room.

Overuse Injuries

Bone   The adolescent with osteochondritis dissecans of the talus may pose a problem to the physician. For example, a child who has sustained an inversion injury to the ankle may have swelling and pain only laterally, without intra-articular swelling. Routine radiographs do not show a definite fracture of the distal fibula, but an area of osteochondritis dissecans of the talus is apparent. The child was asymptomatic before the injury. Do the radiographic findings need further evaluation? Once the osteochondritis dissecans has been recognized, should sports participation be restricted and, if so, for how long? These issues are, for the most part, unsettled.

Sever's disease, or calcaneal apophysitis, is common in 9- to 11-year-old children. The child may have heel pain, particularly when running, and may even be using a tiptoe gait or limping. On physical examination, the calcaneal apophysis is tender to palpation, especially to transverse compression. The Achilles-plantar fascia may be tight. Radiographs are seldom helpful, as the calcaneal apophysis is often fragmented and dense in normal children.

Treatment depends on the severity of the child's symptoms and the degree of the parents' frustration. It is often difficult to control a child's activity levels; for a strongly symptomatic child, a short leg walking cast for ten to 14 days may be the treatment of choice. The cast allows absolute resting of the area. After cast removal and before return to activity, a stretching program must be instituted. For a child who is minimally symptomatic, using a heel lift for several days with a concurrent decrease in running and jumping activities and a stretching program may be all that is required.

Apophysitis at the base of the fifth metatarsal (Ismelin's disease) can occur, but is less common than calcaneal apophysitis. (The proximal epiphysis of the fifth metatarsal usually does not ossify until 15 or 16 years of age.) Symptoms generally respond to a short period of rest.

Soft Tissue   Achilles tendinitis and shin splints occur in the teenager much as they do in the adult. Although adolescents tend to be flexible, some children are not flexible, especially during periods of rapid growth.

Therefore, in the teenager particularly, a flexibility conditioning program should precede and parallel sports participation. Also, if a teenager has symptoms of Achilles tendinitis or shin splint pain, training techniques should be studied to ensure that they are not contributing to the development of the overuse injury. Stair climbing, hill sprinting, toe sprints, and plyometrics may all be reasonable training techniques but should only be used as part of an overall conditioning program and may even need to be eliminated in a youngster with recurrent shin splints or Achilles tendinitis.

Oral nonsteroidal anti-inflammatory drugs are used less frequently in adolescents than in adults, and rarely in children. The preferred treatment uses local anti-inflammatory measures, such as a salicylate cream, ice massage, or physical therapy, combined with a stretching program, heel lifts, arch supports, and taping or strapping.

Sesamoid bursitis—that is, swelling and pain on palpation under the first metatarsal head—is especially likely in sports in which the adolescent "pushes" off the ball of the foot (for example, tennis, racketball) and in dancing on demipoint. Ice massage and salicylate cream coupled with avoidance of the activity for seven to ten days frequently improves symptoms. A full metatarsal arch pad worn in the athlete's regular shoes may also be helpful. A combined metatarsal arch support is better than a simple metatarsal pad for children, because the larger pad may be more effective in decreasing pressure over the first metatarsal head. The pad can be removed after several weeks, when the acute pain has subsided and the swelling about the sesamoid bursa has resolved.

Steroid injections into this area should be avoided. Although injected steroid may give immediate pain relief, it can cause atrophy of the subcutaneous fat and ultimate thinning of the normal protective metatarsal soft tissue pad. The chronic sesamoid bursitis that occurs in adults is rare in children and adolescents.

Impingement syndromes of the ankle do occur, especially in young dancers, gymnasts, and soccer players. In dancers, impingement occurs in the posterior ankle capsule secondary to prolonged maintenance of the plantarflexed position. Symptoms are pain deep to the Achilles tendon, increased by the forced plantarflexion rather than by increased dorsiflexion as in Achilles tendinitis.

Treatment consists of local anti-inflammatory measures to decrease inflammation (ice, salicylate cream, and physical therapy) and avoidance of the marked plantarflexed position until symptoms subside. Strapping a felt pad to the back of the ankle (especially in soccer) may help alleviate the athlete's forced plantarflexed position and prevent impingement.

Fracture of the os trigonum and loose bodies in the posterior aspect of the ankle from chronic impingement are more common in older athletes than in young ones.

The child with an anterior capsular impingement syndrome has acute or gradually increasing pain over the anterior aspect of the ankle. The pain is not associated with intra-articular effusion or with localized swelling in a tendon sheath like that seen in acute tendinitis of the extensor digitorum longus, the extensor digitorum hallucis, or the anterior tibial tendon. In fact, there is often no observable swelling. This syndrome occurs in the gymnast who lands short (that is, lands in marked dorsiflexion) after dismounts or jumps.

Treatment is the same as for posterior capsular impingement—local anti-inflammatory measures and avoidance of the marked flexed position. In anterior capsular impingement syndrome, a pad taped anteriorly over the front of the ankle for several weeks may not only prevent forced impingement during this time but may also give the athlete the "feel" of a correct landing or stance.

Impact of Congenital Variants of Foot and Ankle on Athletic Performance

Congenital skeletal variations of the lower extremities may be undetected until a child puts high demands on the extremities through sports participation.

For example, the young athlete who has a history of multiple ankle sprains and has subtalar stiffness on physical examination may have a previously unrecognized tarsal coalition. Tarsal coalition is also a possible diagnosis for the young athlete with vague intermittent foot pain for several months. The pain is typically aggravated by activity and improved with rest. The age at presentation is usually 8 to 16 years, but can be later. Most cases of tarsal coalition are bilateral. The coalition may be fibrous, cartilaginous, or bony. The most common form is talocalcaneal coalition, followed by calcaneonavicular coalition; calcaneocuboid coalition is the least common. There may be a familial history of the problem as the trait is autosomal dominant with incomplete penetrance.

Calcaneonavicular coalitions are best visualized on a 45-degree oblique view of the foot. A standing lateral radiograph may demonstrate talar beaking, which usually indicates decreased subtalar motion and, hence, is an indirect sign of a tarsal coalition. Many of the coalitions cannot be seen on routine films, and tomography is needed to confirm the suspected diagnosis.

If physical therapy and rest, either by wearing a short leg cast for three to four weeks or using a well-molded orthotic device, does not decrease midfoot pain, or if the child continues to sustain multiple ankle sprains, bar resection can be contemplated. In resection of the calcaneonavicular bar, an adequate amount of material must be excised and the talonavicular joint must be avoided (as cutting the capsule of this joint may result in subluxation of the navicular). Frequently, the extensor digitorum brevis is used as interposition material after resection, so that the bony bridge does not reform. Resection of talocalcaneal bars is more difficult because of the width of the bar.

Children with rigid cavus feet are susceptible to metatarsalgia and "clawing" of their toes. Sorbothane-type padding or custom orthotic devices may be helpful. In athletes with progressive cavus feet, the possibility of neurologic disorders, such as Charcot-Marie-Tooth disease, spinal dysraphism, Friedreich's ataxia, and spinal tumor, must be ruled out.

Barry and Scranton[6] state, "Flat feet in children continue to be

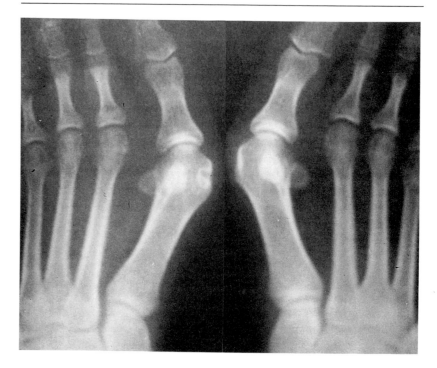

Fig. 5 *Note the increased angle between the first and second metatarsals in this young athlete with adolescent bunions.*

highly overrated and poorly understood." They report that 15% of the population have flat feet. Most cases are asymptomatic. In children with painful flat feet, tarsal coalition or an accessory navicular should be suspected. Accessory naviculars can usually be diagnosed on physical examination, as this extra ossicle is prominent on the medial aspect of the foot. Radiographs confirm the diagnosis. In the symptomatic athlete with an accessory navicular, an orthosis and strengthening of the posterior tibial muscle and the intrinsic muscles of the foot typically diminish symptoms. Surgery is rarely needed.

Adolescent bunions were at one time thought to be caused entirely by improperly fitting shoes. Now, many investigators believe that adolescent bunions result from metatarsus primus varus.[7] The normal angle between the first and second metatarsals is reported to be less than 10 degrees.[8] A child with an angle of more than 10 degrees is likely to develop hallux valgus. There is also a familial tendency to this anatomic variant (Fig. 5).

The deformity itself is not painful if forefoot shoe width is carefully selected to accommodate the widened metatarsal region. However, it is sometimes difficult to find shoes that are stylish but wide enough in the forefoot and narrow enough in the heel to accommodate the foot.

Hallux valgus in the adolescent differs from that in the adult because the degree of valgus of the great toe is usually less. There are no arthritic changes in the metatarsophalangeal joint, and the bursal tissue over the metatarsal head is typically not chronically thickened. Conservative measures, with shoe modification being the prime consideration, are recommended.[7]

Surgical procedures can be done if all conservative measures fail. The surgical procedure decreases the intermetatarsal angle between the first and second metatarsals by either a proximal or distal osteotomy of the first metatarsal. The surgeon must be careful not to alter foot mechanics disadvantageously. The osteotomy should be done with minimal bone loss so that the first metatarsal is not abnormally shortened. This can cause the stress of weightbearing to be transferred to the lesser metatarsal, which may not be strong enough to sustain such forces, thus leading to a stress fracture.

Systemic Diseases and Sports

Systemic diseases must always be considered when sports injuries are diagnosed. Examples include rheumatoid arthritis, acute leukemia, sickle cell trait, and osteogenic sarcoma. The following cases illustrate this point:

(1) A 7-year-old child had sustained an inversion injury to the ankle four weeks earlier. The joint continued to be swollen. When conservative measures failed to decrease the swelling, the joint was aspirated. When the fluid was analyzed, it was found to contain increased protein and to be positive for rheumatoid factor. The diagnosis was rheumatoid arthritis.

(2) Another child had diffuse knee pain that increased during the soccer season. Radiographs were initially noncontributory, but further evaluation because of continued pain resulted in the diagnosis of acute leukemia.

(3) An 11-year-old black child who complained of frequent muscle cramping during sports participation was found to have sickle cell trait.

(4) A teenager complained of persistent leg pain and continued mid-leg swelling after sustaining a blow to the pretibial area in a football game one month earlier. He thought he had only a severe contusion to the area but the diagnosis proved to be osteogenic sarcoma.

References

1. Garrick JG, Requa RK: Injury patterns in children and adolescent skiers. *Am J Sports Med* 1979;7:245-248.
2. Trott AW: Foot and ankle problems in adolescents: Sports aspects. American Academy of Orthopaedic Surgeons *Symposium on Foot and Ankle*, St. Louis, CV Mosby, 1979, p 47.
3. Dias LS: Fractures of the tibia and fibula, in Rockwood CA Jr, Wilkins KE, King RE (eds): *Fractures: Vol 3. Fractures in Children*. Philadelphia, JB Lippincott, 1984, pp 983-1042.

Consensus Statements: Musculoskeletal Injury

1. The public must be educated about the risks for injury in the pediatric age group. This education will result in a mandate for change. Without a sincere desire from parents, officials, and coaches, no change will occur.
2. Past experience and scientific study confirm that rule changes and equipment modification (such as face masks) alter the site and frequency of injury.
3. The identification of pre-existing injury or incomplete rehabilitation of past injury will decrease the occurrence of injury.
4. There is some support for an anatomic predisposition to injury which, if identified, can be used to prevent injury. The scientific documentation is inconclusive, however, so this supposition must be studied further.
5. Controlling the volume and intensity of physical work during sports in this age group will prevent injury.
6. Growth-center injury tends to occur in young athletes, rather than ligamentous and osseous injury seen in adults.

Overuse Syndromes

Chapter 23

Repetitive Stress and
Connective Tissue

Carl L. Stanitski, MD

The term "connective tissue" encompasses a broad range of tissues with variable cell types, cell densities, and cellular metabolic activity. Water, proteoglycan, and collagen contents also vary. Connective tissue acts as a nonlinear, viscoelastic material that is nonisotropic and shows extreme variance in response to macrotrauma and microstresses. The attenuation effects of fatigue and conditioning provide unique models for study.

Most data concerning forces and connective tissue are based on studies of laboratory-induced acute macrostress in adult animals. Few data on the effects of chronic, nondestructive microstress in skeletally immature animals or humans in either laboratory or clinical settings are available.

Sites of connective tissue stress include junctions (bone-muscle, muscle-tendon, tendon-bone, ligament-bone), muscle, tendon, physes, and articular contents. These tissues must be thought of in combination since they do not act as isolated entities.

The effect of growth on connective tissue has received limited attention. The age at onset of the rapid growth phase varies in males and females, as does the rate, magnitude, and duration of growth.

Participation by children and adolescents in sports activities and competitions has increased markedly in the United States. Connective tissue stresses from sports include compression, tension, torsion, shear, and combinations of these. Few data are available on the "normal" features of connective tissues in immature mammalian species. Acute and chronic responses to injuries of varying magnitudes, training techniques, and treatment techniques such as immobilization, graduated stress, and motion sorely need investigation.

Bone-Muscle Junctions

Bone-muscle apophyses at the pelvic brim and spine are vulnerable to both acute and chronic stress. Iliac wing and ischial tuberosity apophyseal avulsions are common manifestations of acute failure at these junctions. Muscle origins along metaphyses and diaphyses of the long bones are common sites of repetitive stress, often manifested by periostitis or muscle tears (commonly known as "shin splints").

Muscle

Muscle is a unique connective tissue. Muscle responds to conditioning by means of cell hypertrophy, fiber splitting, and new cell growth. Significant gains in strength, even in preadolescence, occur with progressive-resistance exercise training. In cats, Giddings and associates[1] noted fiber necrosis with new muscle regeneration of fibers from high-resistance, long-term, concentric exercise. In trained muscle, this muscle-fiber regeneration may account for the hyperplasia and increased strength that occur. Gonyea and associates[2] noted increased numbers of total muscle fibers after exercise in cats and attributed this to fiber splitting. Davies and White[3] commented on diminution of strength in the lower extremities of humans secondary to increased soreness after eccentric load training. After short-term muscle loading in rats that caused muscle strain, Almekinders and Gilbert[4] demonstrated that nonsteroidal anti-inflammatory drugs may inhibit muscle generation. Järvinen and associates,[5] in a study of controlled muscle contusion in rats, showed a diminution in inflammatory response with increasing age. Animals who were not skeletally mature showed a more rapid initial inflammatory reaction with increased ability for phagocytosis compared with more mature animals.

Muscle-Tendon Junctions

The muscle-tendon junction has been considered the "growth plate" of muscle. Crawford[6] initially believed that growth occurred throughout the entire muscle belly. Ziv and associates[7] showed that muscle growth in immature animals is caused by apposition of satellite cells at the muscle-tendon junction, which adds sarcomeres to the end of muscle fibers. Experimental spasticity, which caused a 45% loss of muscle growth, was believed to result from a diminution of a similar proportion in attendant bone. In a study of human tissue, Mair and Tome[8] noted that tendon cellularity is increased at 11 to 18 weeks of fetal development and that the muscle-tendon junction represents a continuity of the muscle fiber, tendon collagen, and sarcolemma. Muscle cells are highly infolded at their interdigitation with tendon. This increase in surface area may allow stress-shielding effects. When growing joints of mice were immobilized, Williams and Goldspink[9] noted a decrease in the normal fiber length of muscles because of a decrease in the number of sarcomeres. When this immobilization was eliminated, sarcomere numbers increased to within the normal range and muscle fiber length was restored to normal within several weeks. To grow normally, muscle must be allowed to contract isotonically. A strict relationship exists among the length of bone, amount of movement, and the number of sarcomeres present.

Tendon

Tendon's properties change with age. Crawford[6] believed that tendon grew throughout its length, with growth greatest at the muscle-tendon junction. Cellular density diminishes after 18 weeks of fetal life and collagen concentration and cross-linking increase as maturity advances. This cross-linking allows for increased energy absorption, as demonstrated in rat tail tendons by Nathan and associates.[10] Significant diminution of vascularity accompanies the reduced cellularity with increased age. Blanten[11] showed that fetal tendon tissue had slightly lower values in tensile-strength testing than human adult tendon tissue. Woo and associates,[12] using swine, showed that increasing amounts of exercise produced increasing tendon strength because of increased cross-sectional area.

Tendon-Bone Junctions

The tendon-bone interface varies with age and as a function of skeletal maturity. This transition zone is a complex junction, with a change from "soft" to "hard" tissue occurring within 1 mm. Benjamin and associates[13] found fibrocartilaginous disk traces in adults and believed that the junction was equivalent to the "tidemark" at the bone-tendon interface in a child. Videman,[14] unlike Crawford, believed that tendons grow most at their insertion site and that newly formed tendon tissue is incorporated directly into osseous tissue. Sharpey's fibers attach periosteum to bone and not to tendon or ligaments. Osteogenesis at the tendon-bone junction allows a smooth mechanical transition from tendon to bone. The serial change of material properties at such junctions provides stress shielding but the area is still a "weak link." Clinical disorders such as Osgood-Schlatter disease, Sinding-Larsen-Johansson disease, and Sever's disease are manifestations of the maturing tendon-bone interface. Sports often cause repetitive microstresses at these tissues, manifested by pain, swelling, and tenderness. Why all such sites are not symptomatic after vigorous exercise is unknown.

Ligaments

Ligaments are specialized connective tissue that provide joint tension, joint surface pressure, and neurofeedback. They are composed primarily of collagen but contain G-actin, myosin, and actin. Ligaments are anisotropic and resist tension along their long axes. The "crimp" in ligaments observed by polarized light microscopy is of questionable significance, but may be related to maturity. If ligament is cyclically loaded to length, peak stresses gradually diminish with time. Clinically, this diminishment may suggest that a warm-up before vigorous and rapid ligament stress should be recommended.

As with other soft tissues, collagen fiber geometry determines mechanical behavior. With increased intermolecular and intramolecular cross-linking, additional age-related changes occur. Cellularity and vascularity diminish with age. Wessels[15] demonstrated in rabbits that growth of approximately 35% occurred throughout all segments of the ligament. This uniform growth is in marked contrast to that noted in muscle, tendon, and bone, which seem to grow at specialized sites. Ligament length remains proportional to physeal growth because of secondary distal ligament fixation that allows retention of the metaphyseal position. Bone-cartilage differentiation during growth allows relative positions of the soft tissues and bones to be maintained. Ligament insertion sites are directly affected by epiphyseal activity and remain structurally inferior until physeal closure. In children, ligament laxity does not occur after epiphysiodesis. The mechanism of such adaptive shortening is unknown.

Frank and associates[16] noted a gradual transitional zone for ligament attachment via fibrocartilage, mineralized fibrocartilage, and then bone. This layered interface allowed stress shielding to occur. Such insertion sites recover slowly from the effects of immobilization because they are fully dependent on bone metabolic activity. In a study by Frank and associates,[17] cell division occurred throughout the ligament but the majority of divisions occurred at the distal metaphyseal attachment area. A structure analogous to periosteum ("periligament") was described by these authors, who believed its function is to add matrix circumferentially to the ligamentous surface.

Ligaments are more than passive structures. Mechanoreceptors in human anterior cruciate ligaments were believed by Schulz and associates[18] to confirm Hinton's law: An afferent arc is present to provide an efferent response to oppose injurious movement.

Ligament strength varies significantly with age and sex. Ligament mechanical properties reach adult values relatively early. The medial collateral ligaments of male and female rats showed no significant difference in resistance to forces of a fixed load.[19] After puberty, however, separation force after a fixed acute load increased in males. When body weight was taken into consideration, female rat medial collateral ligaments were noted to be more resistant to load than male ligaments.

In work done by Peterson and associates[20] on medial collateral ligaments in rabbits, strain rate depended on the entire length of the medial collateral ligament, including the femoral, mid, and tibial complexes. In the immature animal, failure consistently occurred at the junction of the medial collateral ligament and the tibia. After acute load in mature animals, tears consistently occurred within the substance of the ligament and not at the bony attachments. In immature rabbits, Dahners and Muller[21] noted that tension increased the ligament's rate of growth. Under diminished tension, growth continued but at a significantly reduced rate. In a study of immobilization effects on immature rabbit ligaments, Walsh and associates[22] noted diminished cell density after immobilization, but the major effect was decreased secretory activity of ligamentous cells deprived of stress. This secretory function was diminished by as much as 50% to 100% and was inversely proportional to the duration of immobilization. Losses in collagen and plasminogen activator, especially at the end of the ligaments, were found.

Woo and associates,[12] in a study of 1-year-old swine after 12 months of exercise, described an increase in the cross-sectional area of the tendon as well as in cortical bone thickness. No such changes were noted in lateral and medial collateral ligaments. They thought that the exercise model (treadmill running) did not allow valgus and varus stresses adequate to produce physiologic loads on the lateral and medial collateral ligament complex.

When comparing the effect of immobilization with that of progressive exercise, Vailas and associates[23] described significant increases in healing rates in canine medial collateral ligaments resulting from increased collagen synthesis in the exercised group. Studying the effects of exercise on dogs of various ages, Tipton and associates[24] found increased collagen formation in the intact medial collateral ligament along with increased size and number of fibers after intermittent stress exercises on a treadmill.

Epiphysis

The epiphysis is vulnerable during the rapid growth phase of preadolescence. The age at onset and the duration of the rapid growth phase varies in females and males. Shear stress and compressive loads have significant influence on physeal growth. Roy and associates[25] noted significant changes in the distal radial epiphysis of high-level gymnasts. The amount of change was directly related to the intensity of training. After even minor diminutions in intensity, distal radial epiphyseal growth returned to normal. Acute physeal fractures rather than ligament injuries usually occur in the skeletally immature. As skeletons mature, ligament injury becomes more frequent; however, ligament injury in young children is not unknown and is becoming more common as children's sports participation increases.

Articular Contents

Articular contents consist of articular cartilage, meniscal tissue, ligaments, and tendons. Articular cartilage consists primarily of water and shows significant changes in mechanical properties as the dehydration of aging occurs. Loss of permeability also occurs with increasing age and begins a vicious cycle of nutritional deprivation. Failure of the intimate relationship of subchondral structures to articular surfaces was hypothesized as a possible cause of degenerative joint disease by Radin and Rose.[26] Palmoski and Brandt,[27] in a study of histologic changes in canine articular surface after three weeks of cast immobilization, demonstrated that voluntary exercise reversed the histologic effects of immobilization, whereas forced exercise (running 6 miles/day) did not. The negative effects of immobilization were still present after six weeks of such forced exercise.

Buckwalter and associates[28] described significant age-related changes in articular proteoglycans. Clark and Ogden[29] demonstrated that meniscal strength is proportional to age, which is directly related to the meniscal vascularity. The concept of meniscal vascularity has been clinically utilized in meniscal repair.[30]

Summary

In preadolescence and adolescence, marked variability of response to hormonal challenges occurs in both sexes. As with other body tissues, collagen is synthesized and degraded. With increasing age and maturity, significant changes occur in the mechanical properties of connective tissue. Most data on connective-tissue response to injury are based on acute models of surgical and/or mechanical-destructive effects in adult animals. Only a limited amount of data on "normal" connective tissue before skeletal maturity is available; almost no data on the effects of training on connective tissue in skeletally immature humans or laboratory animals exist. Similarly, minimal data are available concerning the repair and regeneration of connective tissue after injury.

A new type of sports injury—the "overuse" injury—is being seen with increasing frequency in the skeletally immature patient. This injury occurs as a consequence of repetitive, nondestructive, submaximal microstresses. The long-term effects of this type of injury remain unknown.

Orthopaedists and others must be reminded that children are not "little adults" either psychologically or physiologically. Attempts to adapt adult orthopaedic reconstruction procedures or sports-training protocols to children do not seem physiologically sound. Much information is needed about the response of connective tissue to acute and chronic stresses in skeletally immature patients.

References

1. Giddings CJ, Neaves WB, Gonyea WJ: Muscle fiber necrosis and regeneration induced by prolonged weight-lifting exercise in the cat. *Anat Rec* 1985;211:133-141.
2. Gonyea W, Ericson GC, Bonde-Petersen F: Skeletal muscle fiber splitting induced by weight-lifting exercise in cats. *Acta Physiol Scand* 1977;99:105-109.
3. Davies CT, White MJ: Muscle weakness following eccentric work in man. *Pflügers Arch* 1981;392:168-171.
4. Almekinders LC, Gilbert JA: Healing of experimental muscle strains and the effects of nonsteroidal anti-inflammatory medication. *Am J Sports Med* 1986;14:303-308.

5. Järvinen M, Aho AJ, Lehto M, et al: Age dependent repair of muscle rupture: A histological and microangiographical study in rats. *Acta Orthop Scand* 1983;54:64-74.

6. Crawford GNC: An experimental study of tendon growth in the rabbit. *J Bone Joint Surg* 1950;32B:234-243.

7. Ziv I, Blackburn N, Rang M, et al: Muscle growth in normal and spastic mice. *Dev Med Child Neurol* 1984;26:94-99

8. Mair WGP, Tome FMS: The ultrastructure of the adult and developing human myotendinous junction. *Acta Neuropathol* 1972;21:239-252.

9. Williams PE, Goldspink G: Longitudinal growth of striated muscle fibres. *J Cell Sci* 1971;9:751-767.

10. Nathan H, Goldgefter L, Kobyliansky E, et al: Energy absorbing capacity of rat tail tendon at various ages. *J Anat* 1978;127:589-593.

11. Blanten B: Mechanical strength of fetal and adult tissue. *J Anat* 1981;223-231.

12. Woo SL-Y, Amiel D, Akeson WH, et al: Effect of long term exercise on ligaments, tendons and bones of swine. *Med Sci Sports Exerc* 1979;11:105.

13. Benjamin M, Evans EJ, Copp L: The histology of tendon attachments to bone in man. *J Anat* 1986;149:89-100.

14. Videman T: An experimental study of the effects of growth on the relationship of tendons and ligaments to bone at the site of diaphyseal insertion. *Acta Orthop Scand* 1970;131(suppl):1-22.

15. Wessels WE, Dahners LE: Growth of the deltoid ligament in the rabbit. *Trans Orthop Res Soc* 1988;13:97.

16. Frank C, Amiel D,Woo SL-Y, et al: Normal ligament properties and ligament healing. *Clin Orthop* 1985;196:15.

17. Frank C, Bodie D, Anderson M, et al: Growth of a ligament. *Trans Orthop Res Soc* 1987;12:42.

18. Schulz RA, Miller DC, Kerr CR, et al: Mechanoreceptors in human cruciate ligaments. *J Bone Joint Surg* 1987;68A:855.

19. Booth FW, Tipton CM: Ligamentous strength measurements in pre-pubescent and pubescent rats. *Growth* 1970;34:177-185.

20. Peterson RH, Gomez MA, Woo SL-Y: The effects of strain rate on the biomechanical properties of the medial collateral ligament: A study of immature and mature rabbits. *Trans Orthop Res Soc* 1987;12:127.

21. Dahners LE, Muller P 22. Walsh S, Frank C, Hart D: Immobilization alters cell function in growing rabbit ligaments. *Trans Orthop Res Soc* 1988;13:57.

23. Vailas AC, Tipton CM, Matthes RD, et al: Physical activity and its influence on the repair process of medial collateral ligaments. *Connect Tissue Res* 1981;9:25-31.

24. Tipton CM, James SL, Mergner W, et al: Influence of exercise on strength of medial collateral knee ligaments of dogs. *Am J Physiol* 1970;218:894-902.

25. Roy S, Caine D, Singer KM: Stress changes of the distal radial epiphysis in young gymnasts: A report of 21 cases and a review of the literature. *Am J Sports Med* 1985;13:301-308.

26. Radin EL, Rose RM: Role of subchondral bone in the initiation and progression of cartilage damage. *Clin Orthop* 1986;213:34-40.

27. Palmoski MJ, Brandt KE: Running inhibits the reversal of atrophic change in canine knee cartilage after removal of a leg cast. *Arthritis Rheum* 1981;24:1329-1336.

28. Buckwalter JA, Kuettner KE, Thonar EJ: Age-related changes in articular cartilage proteoglycans: Electron microscopic studies. *J Orthop Res* 1985;3:251-257.

29. Clark CR, Ogden JA: Development of the menisci of the human knee joint: Morphological changes and their potential role in childhood meniscal injury. *J Bone Joint Surg* 1983;65A:538-547.

30. Arnoczky SP and Warren RF: Microvasculature of the human meniscus. *Am J Sports Med* 1982;10(2):90-95.

Chapter 24

Osteochondroses

Peter D. Pizzutillo, MD

The term osteochondrosis is a substitute for osteochondritis, which denotes an inflammatory or infectious etiology. A host of entities previously grouped under the broad heading of "osteochondroses" have gradually been eliminated from this class by the discovery of their specific causes. These include the endocrinopathies (such as hyperthyroidism), physeal trauma, and changes secondary to the hemoglobinopathies.

The osteochondroses may involve any of the epiphyses and are reported to occur in more than 50 anatomic sites.[1-6] Suggested causes include embolic phenomena, endocrine dysfunction, infection, acute or chronic trauma, hereditary predisposition, and congenital deformity.[1,7-10] Many suggested entities are now recognized as mere radiographic variations of normal ossification of epiphyses without clinical importance and thus are no longer included in this grouping. It is often difficult to differentiate radiographic findings of osteochondroses from normal variations in ossification.[10]

All osteochondroses demonstrate radiographic healing of the defect and relief of symptoms. It has been postulated that all osteochondroses are of uncertain origin and present a clinical pattern of progressive symptoms and a radiographic appearance simulating osteonecrosis.[11] The osteochondroses have been noted to involve previously normal-appearing epiphyses.[10]

Considerable data suggest that normal stress applied to bone in which ossification is delayed may result in the clinical expression of osteochondrosis. When the ossification center of a cartilaginous bone develops late, the child continues to grow in size and may impose unusually increased forces on the developing bony nucleus, producing pain and swelling. Histologically, osteochondroses are characterized by disorderly endochondral ossification of the epiphysis. Most cases occur in the first decade of life and are more common in boys and in the white population.[10]

Certain of the osteochondroses, such as Legg-Calvé-Perthes disease and Kienböck's disease, are avascular in origin. The primary factors that result in an avascular insult have yet to be identified. Osteonecrosis has not been suggested in other osteochondroses because the radiographic appearance does not evolve through the typical phases of destruction and reconstitution seen in osteonecrosis. Instead, there is progressive improvement towards normal ossification and bony morphology.

The following conditions have been grouped according to the classification suggested by Siffert.[12] The primary articular osteochondroses involve the epiphyseal cartilage and the subjacent enchondral ossification, while the secondary articular osteochondroses include ossification centers altered by osteonecrosis. The nonarticular osteochondroses occur at tendon insertions, ligament insertions, or impact sites.[13] The physeal osteochondroses involve physes in the long bones or vertebral bodies.

Articular Osteochondroses

The primary articular osteochondroses include Freiberg's disease and problems involving the humeral condyles, such as Panner's disease.[14]

Freiberg's Disease   Freiberg's disease, first described in 1926, involves collapse of the articular surface and subjacent bone of the metatarsal head[15] (Fig. 1). The second metatarsal head is involved in 68%, the third metatarsal head in 27%, and the fourth metatarsal head in 5% of reported cases.[16] Freiberg's disease results from an avascular insult of unknown cause. Current theories suggest that abnormal stresses delivered to the involved metatarsal head during gait result in microfracture of the subchondral bone, vascular injury, and osteonecrosis.[17] Freiberg's disease is more common in females and is diagnosed most frequently in children 12 to 15 years of age, although it has been reported in patients as young as 10 years of age and in adults.[18] The clinical presentation involves pain in the forefoot on weightbearing or at the extremes of joint motion. Physical examination reveals local tenderness to palpation at the metatarsal head with increased local temperature and occasional swelling.

Nonsurgical treatment is frequently successful in relieving discomfort. Treatment recommendations include restricting activity, using a metatarsal orthotic device, or using a short leg cast with a metatarsal mold. With persistent symptoms, surgical removal of a loose fragment, bone grafting of the metatarsal head, or metatarsal head resection have been reported.[19] Most patients are able to resume running with the use of a relieving metatarsal pad but may still experience pain when jumping.

Complete reossification of the metatarsal head is radiographically apparent after an average of three years. There is permanent distortion of the articular surface. Surgical intervention primarily involves removal of a loose body at the articular surface. Metatarsal head resection has not been successful because painful transfer lesions develop at adjacent metatarsal heads.

Panner's Disease   Panner's disease involves the capitellum of the distal humerus. The average age at diagnosis is 8 years (range, 5 to 10 years);

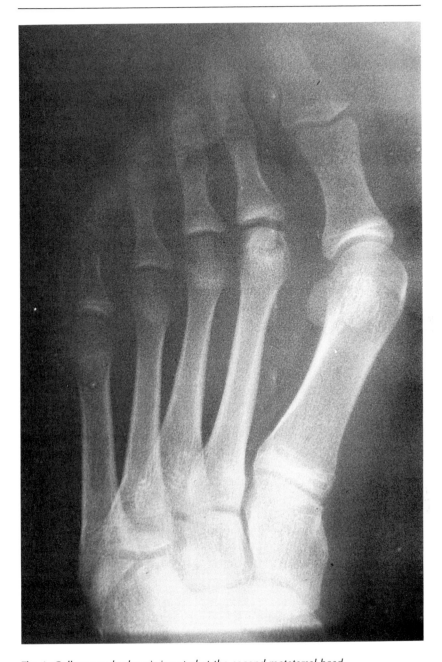

Fig. 1 *Collapse and sclerosis is noted at the second metatarsal head.*

it is more common in boys than in girls.[14] Radiographically, fragmentation and deformity of the ossification center of the capitellum is apparent; progressive reconstitution of the capitellum occurs over a one-to three-year period. Reconstitution occurs with or without therapeutic intervention. The clinical symptoms are pain in the elbow after a trivial injury or an inability to extend the elbow fully.

Treatment includes resting the arm in a sling and avoiding overuse of the involved arm during sports activity.

Osteochondritis Dissecans of the Elbow   Panner's disease should be distinguished from osteochondritis dissecans of the elbow that involves primarily the articular surface and results from osteonecrosis of the subjacent bone. Adams[20] described an injury to the elbow in boys between the ages of 9 and 14 years who had pain and limited range of motion of the elbow. He noted avascular changes involving the medial humeral epiphysis as well as the capitellum and its radial head surface. Woodward and Bianco[21] described bilateral involvement. Elbow pain typically occurs with increased activity and subsides with rest. In addition to an inability to extend the involved elbow fully, complaints include locking, clicking, swelling, and crepitus. Adams[20] compared radiographs of both elbows of 162 athletes (baseball pitchers and nonpitchers) between the ages of 9 and 14 years, and then compared them with radiographs of a control group of nonathletes. He noted significant differences in the pitchers, who demonstrated increased growth and separation of the medial epicondylar epiphysis with fragmentation of the medial epicondylar epiphysis and osteochondritis of the capitellum and the radial head. Flattening of the capitellum and the development of loose bodies may be permanent sequellae. More than half of the patients had enlarged radial heads. Premature closure of the physes of the distal humerus and of the proximal radius has also been documented.[22]

Treatment consists of protected mobilization that generally prohibits full extension of the elbow until radiographic healing is evident. Loose bodies have at times been removed from the elbow in conjunction with curettage and drilling of the base of the defect.[23]

In a review of a slightly older population (average age, 17 years), Grana and Rashkin[24] noted that 42 of 73 pitchers had elbow pain while throwing or developed elbow pain as the season progressed. The symptomatic group had played for a significantly longer period and their radiographs demonstrated asymmetry of the elbow with hypertrophy of the medial epicondyle or of the entire distal humerus.

Secondary Articular Osteochondroses

Legg-Calvé-Perthes Disease   Legg-Calvé-Perthes disease is a condition in which avascular changes develop in the ossification center of the proximal femur. Clinical manifestations generally appear in children 6 to 9 years old but have been reported in children 3 to 12 years old. Perthes' disease is more common in boys and is associated with delayed skeletal maturation. Salter's theory of recurrent ischemic insults leading to osteonecrosis of the subchondral bone and subsequent fracture appears to be most plausible. Patients typically have either a limp or low-grade aching pain in the groin or in the medial aspect of the distal thigh. Physical findings most commonly demonstrate limited abduction and internal rotation of the involved hip compared with the uninvolved hip. Bilateral involvement occurs in 10% of reported cases.

Catterall categorized the extent of involvement of the femoral head in a prognostically significant classification.[25] Catterall type I changes involve decreased bone density at the anterolateral quadrant of the ossification center of the proximal femur, are not associated with collapse, and may be synonymous with so-called Meyer's dysplasia. These changes are not clinically important. In Catterall type II hips, the area of radiographic change is similar to that in type I hips but fragmentation and collapse occur, there is pain, and range of motion becomes limited. Catterall type III hips involve three-fourths of the volume of the proximal ossification center; type IV changes involve the entire femoral head. Both type III and type IV hips are associated with an increased incidence of subsequent hip deformity and poor outcome.

Treatment is controversial and spans the spectrum from benign neglect to surgical intervention. In general, in type I and type II hips, especially in children less than 6 years of age who are symptom-free and maintain a full range of hip motion, observation is indicated. No restriction of athletic activity is indicated. In Catterall type III and type IV hips, even in children less than 6 years of age, the prognosis is guarded (Fig. 2). Without therapeutic intervention to regain a more normal range of hip motion and contain the proximal ossification center of the femur within the acetabulum, many patients will have poor outcomes.[26] The prognosis is worse if the onset of disease occurs after the age of 8 years, especially in girls; by the age of 12 years, the disease is associated with frank migration of the proximal femur out of the acetabulum with subluxation. The femoral head can be contained by traction, physical therapy, or by casting and can be maintained by bracing or surgery such as varus osteotomy of the proximal femur or by innominate osteotomy. No treatment has been uniformly successful. Participation in sports activity can be allowed after reossification of the ossification center of the proximal femur begins, if a brace is used to protect the involved hip.

Osteochondritis Dissecans   Osteochondritis dissecans has received much attention in the orthopaedic literature. Paré removed loose bodies from joints in 1558 and König coined the term osteochondritis dissecans in 1888. The cause is still unknown but suggestions include separation of an abnormal ossification area within an epiphysis, genetic predisposition,[27-30] ischemia,[31] and trauma.[32,33] Repetitive trauma from impact of the tibial spines on the femoral condyle has been suggested as the primary cause of osteochondritis dissecans of the knee. Aichroth[34] noted a high association of knee trauma with the development of osteochondritis dissecans of the knee, but Mubarak and Carroll,[35] in a review of 75 patients, found no relationship between osteochondritis dissecans of

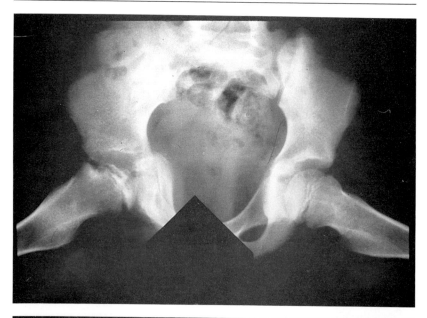

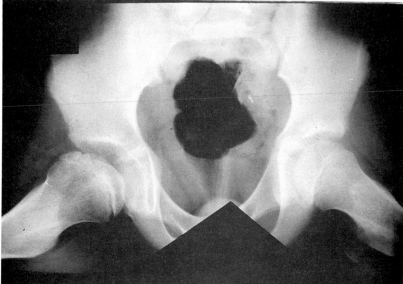

Fig. 2 *Catterall Type IV hip heals with enlargement of the femoral head and mild deformity.*

the knee and trauma, patellar dislocation, or unusually tall tibial spines. Osteochondritic lesions have been created in the canine stifle joint by repeated hyperextension of the joint[33] and in a rabbit joint by excising a small segment of articular cartilage and leaving it attached to synovium. Although ischemia has often been postulated to be a primary cause of osteochondritis dissecans, injection studies have demonstrated a rich blood supply to the femoral condyles.[33] This indicates that ischemia is not likely to be the answer. Possibly osteochondritis dissecans originates as an accessory center of ossification that later separates. Certainly, ossification of the femoral condyles develops in a variety of patterns that have been demonstrated in asymptomatic, normal individuals.

Knee Osteochondritis dissecans of the knee occurs in either the lateral or the medial femoral condyles. The usual age at diagnosis is 13 years (range, 9 to 18 years). Most patients (70%) are male. Mubarak and Carroll[35] reported that 62% of lesions occurred at the lateral aspect of the medial femoral condyle, with 22% at the central portion of the lateral femoral condyle, and 16% in the patella. Multiple lesions including both knees, hips, and elbows are associated with dwarfism[36] and may be inherited.[37]

Green and Banks,[38] Lindén,[39] and Hughston and associates[40] demonstrated that satisfactory healing can be obtained in the knee with open physes by protecting the knee with techniques such as casting[41] (Fig. 3). However, even in the immature knee, if an osteochondral fragment is loose in the joint or partially detached from its base, then surgical treatment (either removal or pin fixation[42] of the fragment with drilling[43] or bone grafting of the base) has been recommended.[44-46] Hughston and associates reported good or excellent results in 82% of those treated nonsurgically and good or excellent results in 77% of those treated surgically. Importantly, their follow-up evaluation found little evidence of degenerative change in knees initially thought to have satisfactory results despite the mode of treatment. VanDemark[47] documented that spontaneous healing of the defect can occur with protected weight-bearing. Smillie[48] emphasized that spontaneous healing, even with protection, does not occur after skeletal maturity.

Femoral Condyle It is difficult to distinguish osteochondritis dissecans of the femoral condyle from an area of irregular ossification.[49] Cahill and Berg[50] reported that technetium phosphate scintigraphy is helpful in the management of juvenile osteochondritis dissecans because clinically important lesions demonstrate an increased uptake during the scanning process, whereas areas of irregular ossification do not.

Talus Osteochondritis dissecans of the talus is similar to osteochondritis dissecans of the knee. Lindén[51] reported an incidence of osteochondritis dissecans of the talus of 0.02 per thousand in both males and females as opposed to an incidence of osteochondritis dissecans of the femoral condyle of 0.6 per thousand in males and 0.3 per thousand in females. The classic work of Berndt and Harty led to the conclusion that osteochondritis dissecans of the talus is traumatic in nature.[52-54] Berndt and Harty[52] correlated clinical material with laboratory models using various amounts of inversion force at the ankle. Their classification is frequently used. Berndt and Harty noted that 43% of lesions were at the middle third of the lateral border of the talus and 57% were in the posterior third of the medial border of the talus. In both adults and

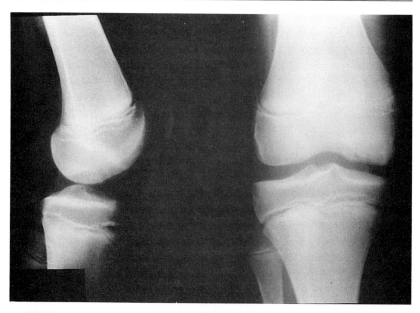

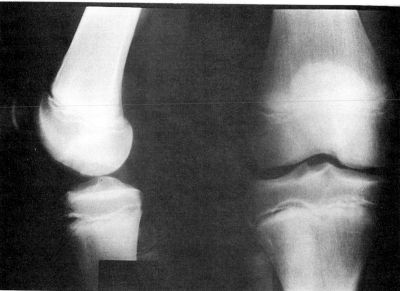

Fig. 3 *Casting has allowed healing of osteochondritis dissecans of the medial femoral condyle in this skeletally immature individual.*

children, results were superior in patients who had been treated surgically rather than nonsurgically.

Canale and Belding[55] and O'Farrell and Costello[56] strongly support a traumatic origin and recommend early surgical treatment. Canale and

Belding did note that arthritic changes in the ankle joint occurred in 50% of patients regardless of treatment. Their specific treatment guidelines were based on the Berndt-Harty classification. Stage I and stage II lesions, that is, those with a nondisplaced fracture within the bony substance, can be treated nonsurgically (Fig. 4). Stage III lesions are fractures through the bone and the cartilage with the fragment remaining within the crater. Those on the medial aspect of the talus can be treated nonsurgically unless symptoms persist. Symptomatic lesions are treated by excision of the lesion and currettage of the base. In stage III lesions of the lateral border of the talus, as well as in all stage IV lesions in which the fragment is completely detached, surgery is recommended.[57-59] A long-term study by Bauer and associates[60] of 30 patients with osteochondritis dissecans of the talus revealed mild radiographic changes and symptoms after an average follow-up of 21 years. Only two of these patients documented arthritic changes. Yuan and associates[61] described two patients with associated subchondral cysts. Seven of the 30 patients included in the study by Bauer and associates had bilateral lesions, suggesting that trauma may not be the sole cause of this problem.[62] Anderson and Lyne[63] reported medial talar lesions in two siblings, neither of whom had associated trauma, endocrinopathy, or abnormal stature.

Köhler's Disease Köhler's disease is a painful condition of childhood involving the tarsal navicular. In 1937 Karp[64] recorded the results of radiographic evaluation of the feet of 25 boys and 25 girls. The evaluation had been repeated every six months from the time the children were 9 months old until they were 4 years old. His studies demonstrated that ossification of the navicular occurred at an earlier age in girls (initial appearance at 18 to 24 months of age in girls compared with 36 months of age in boys). Karp also noted that abnormal ossification centers were more common in centers within the tarsal navicular whose appearance had been delayed. Brower[65] reported that ossification of the tarsal navicular is irregular in 30% of boys and 20% of girls.

The diagnosis of Köhler's disease of the tarsal navicular requires not only the typical radiographic changes of increased density and narrowing in the width of the navicular, but also pain and local tenderness at the navicular. On the basis of vascular injection studies, Waugh[66] postulated that a delay in the appearance of the ossification center in the tarsal navicular may predispose a larger child to this painful disease during normal weightbearing. He believed that abnormal ossification resulted from compression of the bony nucleus at a time during navicular growth when its appearance was significantly delayed.

Williams and Cowell[67] described 23 patients (most of them boys) who began to experience pain between 2 and 9 years of age. All eventually became asymptomatic with total radiographic reconstitution of a normal navicular (Fig. 5). Patients treated with an orthotic device were asymptomatic an average of 15 months after initiation of treatment, whereas patients treated in a cast experienced symptomatic relief after

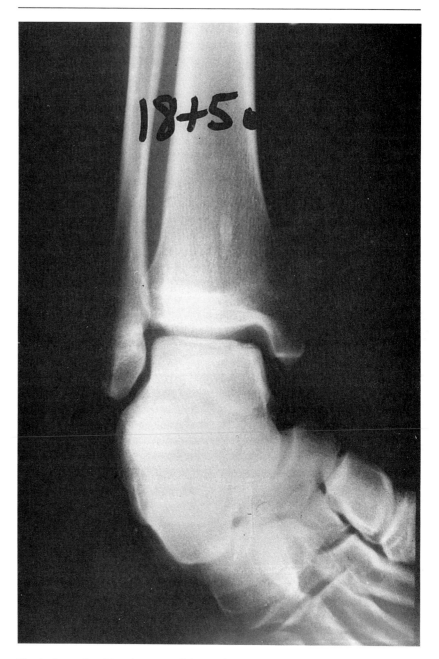

Fig. 4 *Osteochondritis dissecans of the medial border of the talus may remain asymptomatic if the fragment remains nondisplaced.*

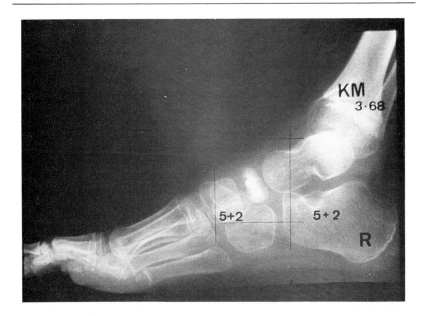

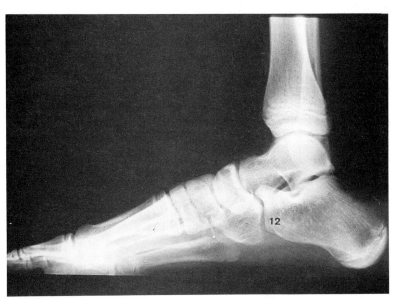

Fig. 5 *Complete reconstitution of Köhler's disease occurs with total resolution of pain.*

an average of 3.2 months. Ippolito and associates[68] reported a long-term evaluation of 12 patients. Their observations were similar to those of Williams and Cowell.

Buschke's Disease Buschke's disease, or osteochondritis of the tarsal cuneiform, is a rare entity[1,69] that involves the medial or middle cuneiform in boys during the first decade of life.[50,70] Pain, the presenting problem, is relieved by rest. Radiographic evaluation reveals eventual total reconstitution of the cuneiform.

Kienböck's Disease   Kienböck's disease is osteonecrosis of the lunate and is more common in the dominant wrist of boys. It is mentioned here for the sake of completeness, but is not considered in depth because it occurs in older patients (20 to 30 years of age).[65]

Nonarticular Osteochondroses

The nonarticular osteochondroses are subdivided into those occurring at a tendon's attachment to bone (for example, Osgood-Schlatter disease), those occurring at a ligament's attachment to bone (for example, at the epicondyles at the elbow or the medial malleolus), and those occurring at impact (for example, at the calcaneus in Sever's disease).

Osgood-Schlatter Disease   Woolfrey and Chandler[71] reported the occurrence of pain and tenderness at the tibial tuberosity in 14- to 15-year-old adolescent boys active in sports (Fig. 6). Ehrenborg[72] concluded that an Osgood-Schlatter lesion was caused by traumatic avulsion of the patellar tendon from the tibial tuberosity. Histologic studies demonstrate an avulsion within the substance of the cartilage of the tibial tubercle.[73] Ehrenborg, in a review of 170 patients, 102 boys and 68 girls, noted bilateral involvement in 28%. The average age at diagnosis was 13 years in boys and 11½ years in girls. After 30 months of follow-up, symptoms had persisted for an average of 27.8 months in knees that had not been immobilized, compared with an average of 14.6 months in knees that had been immobilized.

Ogden and Southwick[74] reviewed various possible causes, including vascular changes, systemic disease, endocrinopathy, structural changes within the tendon substance, and trauma. Histologic findings were consistent with an avulsion of a portion of the developing ossification center with the overlying cartilage. The injury did not involve avulsion through the physeal junction. The histologic evaluation done by Mital and associates[75] demonstrated no signs of osteonecrosis. All fragments were attached to the undersurface of the patellar ligament and were separated from the tubercle by bursal or scar tissue. Kujala and associates[76] reported the results of a questionnaire of 389 adolescents, 193 of whom were active in sports at 13 years of age. They found a history of Osgood-Schlatter disease in 21% of the athletic group but only 4.5% of the nonathletic group. This series reported a 56% incidence of bilaterality.

In children whose knee pain results from direct contact with the tibial tubercle, the problem is usually self-limited and does not require restriction of activity. Contact sports, such as football or soccer, may require the use of a knee pad to protect the tender tibial tubercle. When knee pain occurs during running and jumping in addition to direct

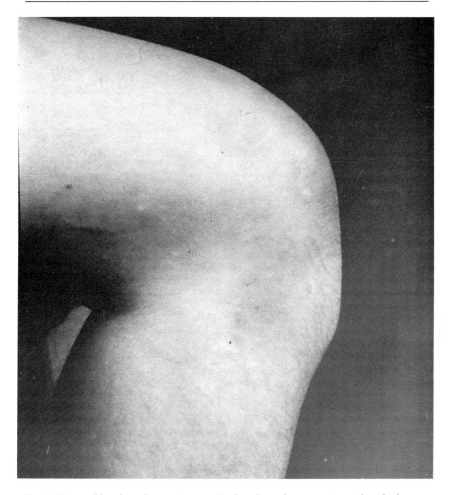

Fig. 6 *Pain and local tenderness is perceived at the enlargement over the tibial tubercle.*

contact, these activities should be restricted for seven to ten days. This usually results in relief of acute symptoms and allows effective rehabilitation of the limb through strengthening exercises.

The complications reported in conjunction with Osgood-Schlatter disease include complete avulsion of the patellar tendon through the anterior aspect of the tibular tubercle and premature fusion of the anterior aspect of the proximal tibial physis with the resultant genu recurvatum.[77,78] Surgical intervention is rarely needed[79] but has been recommended when skeletally mature patients have persistent pain with nonfused ossicles anterior to the tibial tubercle. Simple excision of ossicles has been as successful[80] as the more complicated drilling of the tibial tubercle.[81]

Sinding-Larsen-Johannson Disease   Sinding-Larsen-Johansson disease has also been reported in athletic adolescents who have anterior knee pain.[82] Medlar and Lyne[83] described patients between the ages of 10 and 13 years who complained of pain at the anterior aspect of the knee when running, climbing, or kneeling. There was no history of direct or indirect trauma to the knee and all patients were free of systemic disease. Physical examination demonstrated tenderness to palpation at the inferior pole of the patella, and there was radiographic evidence of fragmentation of the distal pole of the patella. These authors postulated a mechanism of traction tendinitis with calcification in the proximal attachment of the patellar tendon. They described a benign, self-limited clinical course and recommended rest without intervention.

Batten and Menelaus[82] described six 10- and 11-year-old boys with radiographic fragmentation of the proximal pole of the patella. Four of the boys had symptoms of Osgood-Schlatter or Sinding-Larsen-Johansson disease in the same or opposite knee, but none had signs or symptoms relating to the proximal pole of the patella.[82] The other two boys both were asymptomatic. The radiographic appearance of irregular contour of the proximal pole of the patella with loss of the normal trabecular pattern and varying degrees of fragmentation suggests, but does not confirm, partial avulsion of the tendon. A follow-up study of these six boys showed complete resolution of radiographic findings after two years in one patient and significant healing in the others.

Epicondylar Osteochondroses   Involvement at ligamentous attachments to bone is typified by the medial epicondylosis of the distal humerus.[20,84] Boys between the ages of 9 and 14 years may have pain at the medial aspect of the elbow. Many of these patients have played Little League baseball, usually as pitchers. In addition to localized pain at the medial epicondyle of the distal humerus, compression of the ulnar nerve may occur because of repetitive microtears of the arcuate aponeurosis.[85] Radiographs may demonstrate fragmentation of the medial epicondyle with subsequent accelerated growth and associated articular changes at the capitellum. Treatment involves complete rest from throwing activities until healing has occurred and prophylactic measures that limit the number of pitches thrown.

Breck[1] noted that osteochondrosis involving the medial malleolus is rare and is associated with fragmentation and gradual reconstitution. This radiographic finding may be easily confused with an accessory ossification center that frequently occurs at the tip of the medial malleolus.

Sever's Disease   Nonarticular osteochondroses occur at impact sites, such as at the calcaneus in Sever's disease.[86] Micheli and Ireland[87] described 85 children, 52 of whom had bilateral involvement. Most of the children reported that the pain was worse with sports, such as soccer, and all demonstrated weakness of dorsiflexion of the ankle and heelcord contracture. Average age at diagnosis was 11 years 10 months in boys

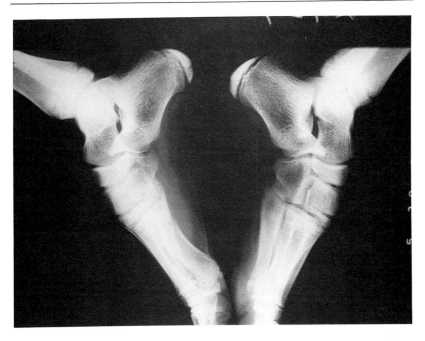

Fig. 7 *Fragmentation and sclerosis of the calcaneal apophysis is seen in normal feet.*

and 8 years 8 months in girls. Sixty-four percent of the patients were boys. Treatment involved heelcord stretching and strengthening of the dorsiflexor of the ankle, as well as the use of inserts or heel cups. After two months, 84 of the patients had improved and were able to resume sports activities. Sever's disease is thought to be secondary to overuse and to stresses imposed by accelerated growth. The radiographic appearance of fragmentation and sclerosis of the calcaneal apophysis is seen in normal, asymptomatic feet and does not indicate Sever's disease (Fig. 7).

Physeal Osteochondroses

Physeal osteochondroses have been reported in long bones (Blount's disease) and in vertebrae (Scheuermann's disease).

Blount's Disease   Blount's disease, or tibia vara, was first described by Elacher in 1922 and later by Blount in 1937,[88] but was characterized by Langenskiöld.[89] Langenskiöld described the typical appearance of the overweight toddler with severe bowing of one or both legs in the first two years of life. He noted that there is an infantile form that begins at walking age and postulated that the adolescent form is a separate entity.

Infantile Tibia Vara Typically, the toddler has an abrupt angulation at the proximal tibia with marked varus of the knee and occasional overgrowth of the distal femur. This is a multidimensional deformity and includes not only varus at the proximal tibia but also internal rotation of the tibia and alteration in the lateral plane of the proximal tibial plateau. Six stages of involvement were defined by radiologic criteria that center about the medial aspect of the proximal tibial physis. Langenskiöld histologically demonstrated islands of densely packed cells with a greater degree of hypertrophy and islands of acellular fibers, cartilage, and large groups of capillary vessels. Typically, the deformity is noted during the second or third year of life with rapid progression occurring during the first four years of life. Gradual spontaneous improvement or static deformity has also been noted. The cause of Blount's disease is still unknown.

Treatment frequently involves early osteotomy of the proximal tibia and fibula as well as osteotomy in combination with epiphysiodesis of the lateral tibial and proximal fibular physes. Complications can result from inadequate correction of the deformity, the need for repeated osteotomy, and neurovascular compromise of the lower leg. Cook and associates[90] reported the results of finite-element analysis of the proximal tibia, and noted that a varus deformity of 30 degrees increased the normal compressive force at the medial tibial physis by a factor of seven. In a 2-year-old child, 20 degrees of varus is sufficient to produce forces that retard physeal growth. In a 5-year-old child, 10 degrees of varus constitutes borderline deformity if the child is of average size but can generate sufficient compressive force in an obese child to inhibit normal growth of the medial half of the proximal tibial physis.

Adolescent Tibia Vara Adolescent tibia vara usually becomes clinically apparent after 9 years of age. The condition tends to be unilateral.[91] Radiographically, the adolescent form differs from the infantile form. In the adolescent form, the radiographic changes primarily involve diminished height of the medial half of the proximal tibial epiphysis without the hooklike medial deformity seen in the infantile form (Fig. 8). Langenskiöld noted that bony bridges at the medial physis can be successfully treated by excision and fat interposition. Wenger and associates[92] reported histologic findings of fissuring and clefts within the substance of the physis with no true bony bridge. In more advanced degrees of deformity or when little growth potential remains in the proximal tibial physis, osteotomy with epiphysiodesis of the lateral half of the proximal tibial physis is indicated.

Individuals with adolescent Blount's disease are frequently very tall and obese. They can participate in most sports, especially wrestling, without increasing the risk of injury as long as there is no ligamentous instability of the knee. The lateral collateral ligament and surrounding soft-tissue complex are subject to continual stress in the presence of significant varus. Once lateral instability of the knee is detected, sports activities must be restricted or bracing must be initiated before a return to activity.

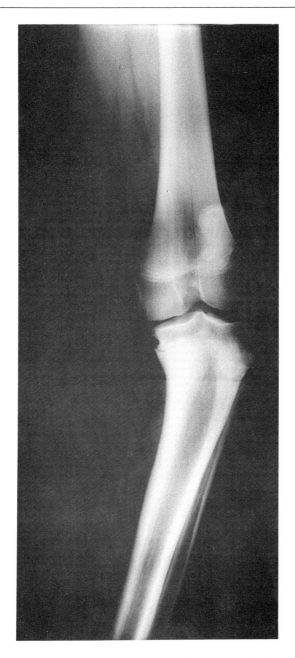

Fig. 8 *Decreased height of the medial portion of the proximal tibial epiphysis is the hallmark of adolescent tibia vara.*

Scheuermann's Disease Scheuermann's disease is a radiographically documented wedge-shaped deformity of one or more vertebrae. The classic criterion of radiographic evidence of three adjacent vertebrae with wedging of 5 degrees or more was proposed by Sorenson.[93] The cause of Scheuermann's disease is not yet known, although many theories have been proposed. Early theories suggested osteonecrosis of the vertebral end plates,[94] but histologic specimens obtained at the time of surgery failed to demonstrate avascular changes.[95] Longitudinal growth of the vertebral body occurs at the superior and the inferior growth plates of the vertebral body with no contribution to longitudinal growth by the ring apophyses. Radiography reveals irregularities of the end plates, narrowing of the disk spaces, increased thoracic kyphosis, and at least 5 degrees of vertebral wedging. When the increased kyphosis is in the thoracic spine, there is a concomitant increase in lumbar lordosis. When dorsal-lumbar kyphosis occurs, there is flattening of the lumbar lordosis with a secondary lordotic deformity above the kyphosis into the thoracic spine. Radiographic studies of lumbar Scheuermann's disease reveal an increased anteroposterior diameter of the vertebral bodies compared with the vertebrae above or below the involved segments. Large lucent defects appear in either the anterosuperior or anteroinferior borders of the vertebral bodies (Fig. 9). Lumbar Scheuermann's disease has a significantly higher association with low back pain than does thoracic Scheuermann's disease.

The pathogenesis of Scheuermann's disease was investigated by Aufdermaur and Spycher,[96] who demonstrated loosening or interruption of the collagen fibers in the end plates of the vertebral bodies. They thought that a disturbance in collagen biosynthesis might cause this problem. Bradford[97] suggested a process similar to idiopathic juvenile osteoporosis as the primary cause in the production of Scheuermann's kyphosis. Kozlowski and Middleton[98] suggested that lumbar Scheuermann's disease is essentially the result of anterior disk herniation in the immature spine.

Treatment of Scheuermann's kyphosis depends on the existence of back pain, neurologic compromise, or cosmetic concerns.[99,100] Dorsal kyphosis of less than 50 degrees is rarely symptomatic or of cosmetic concern. When kyphosis exceeds 50 degrees, however, patients may complain of back pain and the appearance of the compensatory hyperlordosis at the lumbar spine and at the cervical spine. Neurologic compromise is not common in Scheuermann's disease but has been reported. When a child or adolescent has a kyphotic curve in excess of 50 degrees that is supple enough to reduce to normal ranges by hyperextension, then bracing and exercises may be treatment options. In the presence of fixed deformity, surgical treatment requires anterior release of the anterior longitudinal ligament and resection of the disks, followed by posterior stabilization and correction of the deformity with compression Harrington rods and bone grafting. Lumbar Scheuermann's disease may be improved with the use of bracing; however, complete reconstitution of normal dorsal kyphosis and lumbar lordosis is rarely attained.

Athletes with Scheuermann's disease may participate in many sports activities, including contact sports, as long as they are not involved in brace treatment. Once brace treatment has been initiated, only non-

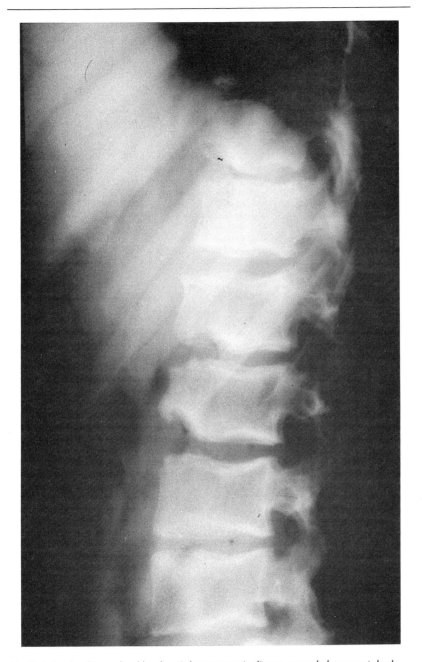

Fig. 9 *Lateral radiograph of lumbar Scheuermann's disease reveals large vertebral bodies with defects noted at anterosuperior or anteroinferior borders of the body.*

contact sports should be allowed. Weightlifting activities should also be restricted while the patient is in active treatment, although low-resistance exercise with multiple repetitions, as well as bench-pressing exercises, are well tolerated.

References

1. Breck LW: *An Atlas of the Osteochondroses.* Springfield, Charles C Thomas, 1971.
2. Byers PD: Ischio-pubic osteochondritis: Report of a case and a review. *J Bone Joint Surg* 1963;45B:694-702.
3. Durham HA: Ischiopubic osteochondritis. *J Bone Joint Surg* 1937;19:937-944.
4. Hall TD: Osteochondritis of the greater trochanteric epiphysis. *J Bone Joint Surg* 1958;40A:644-646.
5. Hassler WL, Heyman CH, Bennett JW: Osteochondritis of the distal tibial epiphysis: A report of two cases. *J Bone Joint Surg* 1960;42A:1261-1264.
6. Schmier AA, Meyers MP: Bilateral osteochondritis of the pisiform bones: Report of a case. *J Bone Joint Surg* 1939;21:789-791.
7. Douglas G, Rang M: The role of trauma in the pathogenesis of the osteochondroses. *Clin Orthop* 1981;158:28-32.
8. Duthie RB, Houghton GR: Constitutional aspects of the osteochondroses. *Clin Orthop* 1981;158:19-27.
9. Mau H: Juvenile osteochondroses: Enchondral dysostoses. *Clin Orthop* 1958; 11:154-167.
10. Siffert RS: The osteochondroses. *Clin Orthop* 1981;158:2-3.
11. Taglialavoro G, Ferrari GP, Turra S: Osteochondritis dissecans of the talus: A report on seven cases. *Ital J Orthop Traumatol* 1985;11:301-308.
12. Siffert RS: Classification of the osteochondroses. *Clin Orthop* 1981;158:10-18.
13. Katz JF: Nonarticular osteochondroses. *Clin Orthop* 1981;158:70-76.
14. Omer GE Jr: Primary articular osteochondroses. *Clin Orthop* 1981;158:33-40.
15. Freiberg AH: So-called infraction of the second metatarsal bone. *J Bone Joint Surg* 1926;8:257-261.
16. Binek R, Levisohn EM, Bersani F, et al: Freiberg disease complicating unrelated trauma. *Orthopedics* 1988;11:753-757.
17. Braddock GTF: Experimental epiphysial injury and Freiberg's disease. *J Bone Joint Surg* 1959;41B:154-159.
18. Smillie IS: Freiberg's infraction (Köhler's second disease). *J Bone Joint Surg* 1957;39B:580.
19. Gauthier G, Elbaz R: Frieberg's infraction: A subchondral bone fatigue fracture. A new surgical treatment. *Clin Orthop* 1979;142:93-95.
20. Adams JE: Bone injuries in very young athletes. *Clin Orthop* 1968;58:129-140.
21. Woodward AH, Bianco AJ Jr: Osteochondritis dissecans of the elbow. *Clin Orthop* 1975;110:35-41.
22. Roberts N, Hughes R: Osteochondritis dissecans of the elbow joint: A clinical study. *J Bone Joint Surg* 1950;32B:348-360.
23. McManama GB Jr, Micheli LJ, Berry MV, et al: The surgical treatment of osteochondritis of the capitellum. *Am J Sports Med* 1985;13:11-21.
24. Grana WA, Rashkin A: Pitcher's elbow in adolescents. *Am J Sports Med* 1980;8:333-336.
25. Catterall A: The natural history of Perthes' disease. *J Bone Joint Surg* 1971; 53B:37-53.
26. MacEwen GD: Treatment of Legg-Calvé-Perthes Disease, in Murray DG (ed): American Academy of Orthopaedic Surgeons *Instructional Course Lectures,* XXX. St. Louis, CV Mosby, 1981, pp 75-84.

27. Andrew TA, Spivey J, Lindebaum RH: Familial osteochondritis dissecans and dwarfism. *Acta Orthop Scand* 1981;52:519-523.

28. Auld CD, Chesney RB: Familial osteochondritis dissecans and carpal tunnel syndrome. *Acta Orthop Scand* 1979;50:727-730.

29. Gardiner TB: Osteochondritis dissecans in three members of one family. *J Bone Joint Surg* 1955;37B:139-141.

30. Hay BM: Two cases of osteochondritis dissecans affecting several joints. *J Bone Joint Surg* 1950;32B:361-367.

31. Pappas AM: Osteochondrosis dissecans. *Clin Orthop* 1981;158:59-69.

32. Campbell CJ, Ranawat CS: Osteochondritis dissecans: The question of etiology. *J Trauma* 1966;6:201-221.

33. Clanton TO; DeLee JC: Osteochondrosis dissecans: History, pathophysiology and current treatment concepts. *Clin Orthop* 1982;67:50-64.

34. Aichroth P: Osteochondritis dissecans of the knee: A clinical survey. *J Bone Joint Surg* 1971;53B:440-447.

35. Mubarak SJ Carroll NC: Juvenile osteochondritis dissecans of the knee: Etiology. *Clin Orthop* 1981;157:200-211.

36. White J: Osteochondritis dissecans in association with dwarfism. *J Bone Joint Surg* 1957;39B:261-267.

37. Mubarak SJ, Carroll NC: Familial osteochondritis dissecans of the knee. *Clin Orthop* 1979;140:131-136.

38. Green WT, Banks HH: Osteochondritis dissecans in children. *J Bone Joint Surg* 1953;35A:26-47.

39. Lindén B: Osteochondritis dissecans of the femoral condyles: A long-term follow-up study. *J Bone Joint Surg* 1977;59A:769-776.

40. Hughston JC, Hergenroeder PT, Courtenay BG: Osteochondritis dissecans of the femoral condyles. *J Bone Joint Surg* 1984;66A:1340-1348.

41. Outerbridge RE: Osteochondritis dissecans of the posterior femoral condyle. *Clin Orthop* 1983;175:121-129.

42. Lindholm S, Pylkkänen P: Internal fixation of the fragment of osteochondritis dissecans in the knee by means of bone pins: A preliminary report on several cases. *Acta Chir Scand* 1974;140:626-629.

43. Gepstein R, Conforty B, Weiss RE, et al: Closed percutaneous drilling for osteochondritis dissecans of the talus: A report of two cases. *Clin Orthop* 1986;213:197-200.

44. Cahill B: Treatment of juvenile osteochondritis dissecans and osteochondritis dissecans of the knee. *Clin Sports Med* 1985;4:367-384.

45. Lee CK, Mercurio C: Operative treatment of osteochondritis dissecans in situ by retrograde drilling and cancellous bone graft: A preliminary report. *Clin Orthop* 1981;158:129-136.

46. Lindholm TS, Osterman K: Treatment of juvenile osteochondritis dissecans of the knee. *Acta Orthop Belg* 1979;45:643.

47. VanDemark RE: Osteochondritis dissecans with "spontaneous healing." *J Bone Joint Surg* 1952;34A:143-148.

48. Smillie IS: Treatment of osteochondritis dissecans. *J Bone Joint Surg* 1957;39B:248-260.

49. Langer F, Percy EC: Osteochondritis dissecans and anomalous centres of ossification: A review of 80 lesions in 61 patients. *Can J Surg* 1971;14:208-215.

50. Cahill BR, Berg BC: 99m-Technetium phosphate compound joint scintigraphy in the management of juvenile osteochondritis dissecans of the femoral condyles. *Am J Sports Med* 1983;11:329-335.

51. Lindén B: The incidence of osteochondritis dissecans in the condyles of the femur. *Acta Orthop Scand* 1976;47:664-667.

52. Berndt AL, Harty M: Transchondral fractures (osteochondritis dissecans) of the talus. *J Bone Joint Surg* 1959;41A:988-1020.

53. Cameron BM: Osteochondritis dissecans of the ankle joint: Report of a case simulating a fracture of the talus. *J Bone Joint Surg* 1956;38A:857-861.

54. Mukherjee SK, Young AB: Dome fracture of the talus: A report of ten cases. *J Bone Joint Surg* 1973;55B:319-326.

55. Canale ST, Belding RH: Osteochondral lesions of the talus. *J Bone Joint Surg* 1980;62A:97-102.

56. O'Farrell TA, Costello BG: Osteochondritis dissecans of the talus: The late result of surgical treatment. *J Bone Joint Surg* 1982;64B:494-497.

57. Alexander AH, Lichtman DM: Surgical treatment of transchondral talar-dome fractures (osteochondritis dissecans): Long-term follow-up. *J Bone Joint Surg* 1980;62A:646-652.

58. Baker CL, Andrews JR, Ryan JB: Arthroscopic treatment of transchondral talar-dome fractures. *Arthroscopy* 1986;2:82-87.

59. Thompson JP, Loomer RL: Osteochondral lesions of the talus in a sports medicine clinic: A new radiographic technique and surgical approach. *Am J Sports Med* 1984;12:460-463.

60. Bauer M, Johnson K, Lindén B: Osteochondritis dissecans of the ankle: A 20-year follow-up study. *J Bone Joint Surg* 1987;69B:93-96.

61. Yuan HA, Cady RB, DeRosa C: Osteochondritis dissecans of the talus associated with subchondral cysts: Report of three cases. *J Bone Joint Surg* 1979;61A:1249-1251.

62. McCullough CJ, Venugopal V: Osteochondritis dissecans of the talus: The natural history. *Clin Orthop* 1979;144:264-268.

63. Anderson DV, Lyne ED: Osteochondritis dissecans of the talus: Case report on two family members. *J Pediatr Orthop* 1984;4:356-357.

64. Karp MG: Köhler's disease of the tarsal scaphoid: End-result study. *J Bone Joint Surg* 1937;19:84-96.

65. Brower AC: The osteochondroses. *Orthop Clin North Am* 1983;14:99- 117.

66. Waugh W: The ossification and vascularization of the tarsal navicular and their relation to Köhler's disease. *J Bone Joint Surg* 1958;40B:765-777.

67. Williams GA, Cowell HR: Köhler's disease of the tarsal navicular. *Clin Orthop* 1981;158:53-58.

68. Ippolito E, Ricciari-Pollini PT, Falez' F: Köhler's disease of the tarsal navicular: Long-term follow-up of 12 cases. *J Pediatr Orthop* 1984;4:416-417.

69. Leeson MC, Weiner DS: Osteochondrosis of the tarsal cuneiforms. *Clin Orthop* 1985;196:260-264.

70. Zimberg J, Levitt JC, Brahim F: Osteochondrosis of the medial cuneiform: A case report. *J Am Podiatr Med Assoc* 1985;75:538-539.

71. Woolfrey BF, Chandler EF: Manifestations of Osgood-Schlatter's disease in late teen age and early adulthood. *J Bone Joint Surg* 1960;43A:327-332.

72. Ehrenborg G: The Osgood-Schlatter lesion: A clinical study of 170 cases. *Acta Chir Scand* 1962;124:89-105.

73. Ehrenborg G, Engfeldt B: Histologic changes in the Osgood-Schlatter lesion. *Acta Chir Scand* 1961;121:328-337.

74. Ogden JA, Southwick WO: Osgood-Schlatter's disease and tibial tuberosity development. *Clin Orthop* 1976;116:180-189.

75. Mital MA, Matza RA, Cohen J: The so-called unresolved Osgood-Schlatter lesion: A concept based on 15 surgically treated lesions. *J Bone Joint Surg* 1980;62A:732-739.

76. Kujala UM, Kvist M, Heinonen O: Osgood-Schlatter's disease in adolescent athletes: Retrospective study of incidence and duration. *Am J Sport Med* 1985; 13:236-241.

77. Jeffreys TE: Genu recurvatum after Osgood-Schlatter's disease: Report of a case. *J Bone Joint Surg* 1965;47B:298-299.

78. Stirling RI: Complications of Osgood-Schlatter's disease. *J Bone Joint Surg* 1952;34B:149-150.

79. Thompson JEM: Operative treatment of osteochondritis of the tibial tubercle. *J Bone Joint Surg* 1956;38A:142-148.

80. Glynn MK, Regan BF: Surgical treatment of Osgood-Schlatter's disease. *J Pediatr Orthop* 1983;3:216-219.

81. Hucherson DC, Claussen BF: Osgood-Schlatter's disease: Perforation of the tibial tubercle. *Am J Orthop* 1960;2:198.

82. Batten J, Menelaus MB: Fragmentation of the proximal pole of the patella: Another manifestation of juvenile traction osteochondritis. *J Bone Joint Surg* 1985; 67B:249-251.

83. Medlar RC, Lyne ED: Sinding-Larsen-Johansson disease: Its etiology and natural history. *J Bone Joint Surg* 1978;60A:1113-1116.

84. Singer KM, Roy SP: Osteochondrosis of the humeral capitellum. *Am J Sports Med* 1984;12:351-360.

85. Hang YS: Tardy ulnar neuritis in a Little League baseball player. *Am J Sports Med* 1981;8:244-246.

86. Sever JW: Apophysitis of the os calcis. *NY Med J* 1912;95:1025-1029.

87. Micheli LJ, Ireland ML: Prevention and management of calcaneal apophysitis in children: An overuse syndrome. *J Pediatr Orthop* 1987;7:34-38.

88. Blount WP: Tibia vara, osteochondrosis deformans tibiae. *Curr Pract Orthop Surg* 1966;3:141-156.

89. Langenskiöld A: Tibia vara: Osteochondrosis deformans tibiae: Blount's disease. *Clin Orthop* 1981;158:77-82.

90. Cook SD, Lavernia CJ, Burke SW, et al: A biomechanical analysis of the etiology of tibia vara. *J Pediatr Orthop* 1983;3:449-454.

91. Thompson GH, Carter JR, Smith CW: Late-onset tibia vara: A comparative analysis. *J Pediatr Orthop* 1984;4:185-194.

92. Wenger DR, Mickelson M, Maynard JA: The evolution and histopathology of adolescent tibia vara. *J Pediatr Orthop* 1984;4:78-88.

93. Sorenson HK: *Scheuermann's Juvenile Kyphosis.* Munksgaard, Copenhagen, 1964.

94. Buchman J: Osteochondritis of the vertebral body. *J Bone Joint Surg* 1927;9:55-66.

95. Ippolito E, Ponseti IV: Juvenile kyphosis: Histological and histochemical studies. *J Bone Joint Surg* 1981;63A:175-182.

96. Aufdermaur M, Spycher M: Pathogenesis of osteochondrosis juvenilis Scheuermann. *J Orthop Res* 1986;4:452-457.

97. Bradford DS: Vertebral osteochondrosis (Scheuermann's kyphosis). *Clin Orthop* 1981;158:83-90.

98. Kozlowski K, Middleton R: Familial osteochondritis dissecans: A dysplasia of articular cartilage? *Skel Radiol* 1985;13:207-210.

99. Bradford DS, Ahmed KB, Moe JH, et al: The surgical management of patients with Scheuermann's disease: A review of 24 cases managed by combined anterior and posterior spine fusion. *J Bone Joint Surg* 1980;62A:705-712.

100. Bradford DS, Moe JH, Montalvo FJ, et al: Scheuermann's kyphosis. *J Bone Joint Surg* 1975;57A:439-448.

Chapter 25

Stress Fractures in the Pediatric Athlete

D. A. Yngve, MD

Epidemiology

Stress fractures occur in children less frequently than in adolescents or adults. A recent study[1] of 368 stress fractures revealed that 9% occurred in children 15 years old or younger, 32% occurred in adolescents 16 to 19 years old, and 59% occurred in adults 20 years of age and older.

A review of 23 published reports revealed 131 stress fractures in children under 14 years old. Many reports involved only a single case or a small number of cases. There is a difference between pediatric athletes and adult athletes in the distribution of stress fractures throughout the body. In 94 pediatric cases, the bone involved was identified. The tibia was involved in 51% of these fractures,[2-7] the fibula in 20%,[3,8] and the femur in 3%.[5,7] Defects in the pars interarticularis occurred in 15% of the cases.[9,10] There were two reports of metatarsal involvement,[3] two of tarsal navicular involvement,[11,12] and two of ulnar involvement.[13,14] Single cases of fractures of the humerus,[15] patella,[16] first rib, and medial sesamoid bone[3] were reported.

In two large series of stress fractures in adult athletes,[1,17] the tibia was involved in 50%, almost the same as the pediatric incidence of 51%. However, metatarsal involvement was more common (14% in adults compared with 2% in children) and spinal involvement was less common (less than 1% in adults compared with 15% in children).

Etiology and Prevention

Stress fractures most often result from abnormal stresses on normal bone. However, normal stresses on abnormal bone can also produce stress fractures. Bone diseases such as osteogenesis imperfecta, metabolic disorders such as rickets, neurologic disorders such as myelomeningocele and paraplegia, and other conditions such as postirradiation changes can decrease the resistance of a bone to stress fracture.[18] The anatomic configuration of a bone can also determine its mechanical resistance to stress fracture. Milgrom and associates[19] found that the incidence of tibial stress fractures among Israeli recruits correlated with tibial bending strength. Anteroposterior and lateral tibial radiographs of the recruits were obtained prospectively. Theoretical bending strengths were calculated in the frontal and sagittal planes. The 20% who later developed stress fractures of the tibia, all of which occurred along the medial tibial cortex, had decreased tibial bending strengths in the frontal plane.

Experimental work has shown that a new loading regimen must last longer than two weeks before the bone responds with increased strength. In an experimental study of in vivo rooster ulnas, bone mineral content was monitored with single-photon densitometry while the ulnas were stressed in a controlled fashion. There was no increase in bone mineral content during the first two weeks of loading but there was a rapid increase during the third and fourth weeks. Histologic studies showed that the primary increase in bone mineral content was caused by periosteal and endosteal new-bone formation.[20] It should be noted that this experimental model used an essentially nonweightbearing bone.

The same principle was demonstrated in humans in a prospective study that modified the training of military recruits. One group of recruits underwent a modified basic training program in which running, jumping, and double-timing were eliminated during the third week of training. A second group underwent a conventional training program that continued these activities during the third week. The stress fracture rate was 4.8% in the group with conventional training and only 1.6% in the group with modified training. The final performance test scores were equal. Thus, eliminating the running, jumping, and double-timing during the third week substantially reduced the stress fracture rate.[21]

These two studies demonstrate the principle of skeletal conditioning. When increased loading is applied to a bone, its strength does not start to increase until after the 14th day. If loading is kept constant, the bone continues to increase in strength from the 14th to the 28th day.[20]

Muscle strength can increase faster than bone strength. Muscle strength can increase within two weeks of the onset of a training program. An athlete two weeks into a training program could have an imbalance of muscle and bone strength, as the bone would not yet have responded. Early muscle strength gains may be the result of neural factors because muscle hypertrophy does not become a significant factor in increased strength until after the third week.[22]

These principles underlie the primary training error that leads to stress fractures—doing too much too soon. Other factors that may contribute to stress fractures are running on excessively hard training surfaces and wearing shoes with inadequate shock-absorbing properties.[1] Hormonal factors may also play a role. An increased incidence of stress fractures was reported in ballet dancers (18 to 36 years old) who were older than average at menarche.[23]

Diagnosis and Treatment

Stress fractures must be distinguished from other overuse injuries such as tendinitis, ligament sprains, and contusions. Plain radiographs alone should provide the diagnosis in about 50% of stress fractures, although the radiographic findings may be subtle. When a stress fracture occurs in cancellous bone, a radiolucent fracture line is most commonly seen. In cortical bone, cortical thickening may be the only sign. Radiographs are not often helpful during the first two weeks.

In cases in which radiographs are not conclusive, bone scintigraphy is recommended. Bone scintigraphy misses very few lesions and is extremely helpful in diagnosing stress fractures. However, not every area of increased bone uptake represents a stress fracture. Inflammatory processes, ligamentous avulsion injuries, and tumors may produce abnormal bone images that resemble stress fractures.[11] Subclinical stress fractures, called stress reactions, are commonly found by bone scintigraphy. Stress reactions are areas of bone remodeling that usually remain asymptomatic and resolve in several weeks.

Rest is the usual treatment for stress fractures. In many cases, general conditioning can be maintained during recovery by exercising other areas of the body or by continuing the same activities with less intensity. Stress fractures occasionally develop into displaced fractures when the warning symptoms are ignored.[14]

Stress fractures of the tibial shaft are resistant to treatment and can persist for more than a year. Electrical stimulation may be indicated for these fractures.[4] Some stress fractures of the pars interarticularis have healed when treated by immobilization. Methods of immobilization have ranged from a pantaloon spica cast to a corset.[10]

Specific Sports

Of the 131 cases of pediatric stress fractures reported in the literature, 34 were sports-related. Running was involved the most frequently with eight cases (24%), and gymnastics was second with seven cases (21%). Ice skating was involved in five cases (15%), basketball in four cases (13%), football in three cases (9%), and baseball in two cases (6%). There was one reported case each for soccer, swimming, tennis, and volleyball. As would be expected, the injury sites were strongly sports-related.

Running   Of the eight stress fractures related to running, six involved the tibia, one the tarsal navicular, and one the distal femur. Sites of tibial involvement can be the proximal or distal metaphysis or the midshaft. The fracture site was specified in four cases: three were proximal metaphyseal and one was distal metaphyseal.

Gymnastics   Of the seven stress fractures associated with gymnastics, all involved the pars. In a study of 100 young female gymnasts, an 11%

incidence of pars defects was found. This is about four times the 2.3% incidence in the general female population.[9] The symptoms were characterized by a chronic, dull, aching pain, usually of insidious onset, and aggravated by hyperextension, like that occurring during back walkovers. Jackson and associates[9] believed that to ignore the early symptoms increases the risks of developing pars defects.[9] Probably, too little is known about the causes of pars defects to be able to make specific recommendations for prevention. Back hyperextension may be related, but dismounts performed with the body stiffly extended may also be responsible.[24,25] Early diagnosis is important. If plain radiographs are noncontributory, bone scintigraphy may help in making the diagnosis. Immobilization is recommended for acute injuries.[10]

Ice Skating   Ice skating characteristically causes a stress fracture of the distal fibula. This fracture occurs with eversion of the foot in beginning skaters. Eversion forces can become magnified when skates are worn because the blade of the skate raises the foot off the ice.[8]

Basketball   Of the four stress fractures related to basketball, three were of the tibia and one was of the tarsal navicular. One of the three tibial fractures involved the anterior cortex of the midshaft. This patient had symptoms for 12 months before treatment and healed after six months of treatment with pulsed electromagnetic fields, when a return to activity was allowed.[4]

Football   Of the three stress fractures related to football, all involved the pars. Typically, the players had had some backache and muscle spasms all season. One particular incident then caused the symptoms to intensify. The most likely explanation of this phenomenon is that a stress fracture was developing when the particular incident caused a complete separation of the bone fragments.[10]

Adult interior linemen have been reported to have a 24% incidence of spondylolysis, which is much higher than the 6.4% incidence in white men and 2.8% incidence in black men.[26] It has been postulated that the three-point stance with hyperextension of the lumbosacral spine creates abnormal forces on the posterior elements, particularly when blocking with force.[27]

Baseball   Of the two stress fractures related to baseball, one involved the tibia[6] and one involved the humerus.[15] The stress fracture of the humerus developed into a complete fracture. The patient was a 13-year-old Little League pitcher with a one-week history of aching in the area of the humerus at rest and during pitching. His specialty was a forceful sidearm curve ball pitch that he used exclusively, despite warnings from his coach and local umpires. During one forceful pitch, the humerus snapped with an audible crack. It healed after treatment with immobilization. The patient listened to suggestions and altered his pitching style after this episode.[15]

Soccer   One case of stress fracture of the patella has been reported in a soccer player. The patient had had six months of patellar pain. The pain intensified when he kicked a ball. Radiographs revealed a nondisplaced transverse fracture of the patella.[16]

Swimming   A stress fracture of the proximal tibia was reported in an 8-year-old swimmer who specialized in the breast stroke. She had increased swimming practice to about five hours a day when the symptoms developed. The patient was successfully treated with activity restriction.[28]

Tennis   A stress fracture of the left ulna was reported in a right-handed tennis player. This player used the left hand for two-handed back-hand shots.[14]

Volleyball   A stress fracture in the midshaft ulna was reported in the dominant arm of a volleyball player. The fracture healed with activity restriction.[13]

Summary

The most characteristic difference between adult and pediatric stress fractures is the high prevalence of stress fractures of the pars in the pediatric group. In gymnasts and interior linemen on football teams, the incidence is about four times that in the general population. The causes have not been clearly delineated; however, hyperextension and high axial loading have been implicated. Usually, these stress fractures are preceded by premonitory symptoms. Continued participation in gymnastics or football despite aching in the low back may lead to a pars fracture.

Paying attention to symptoms is important. A runner with persistent pain in the proximal metaphyseal area of the tibia might be advised to modify the training program to control symptoms, since the proximal tibia is a common location for tibial stress fractures in pediatric runners.

The principle of bone conditioning is to stress the bone for a two-week period and then to allow it to strengthen itself for the next one to two weeks. This principle should be kept in mind when designing training programs. It can be carried out by cutting back on training intensity during the third week.

References

1. Hulkko A, Orava S: Stress fractures in athletes. *Int J Sports Med* 1987;8:221-226.
2. Daffner RH, Salutario M, Gehweiler JA, et al: Stress fractures of the proximal tibia in runners. *Diag Radiol* 1982;142:63-65.
3. Devas MB: Stress fractures in children. *J Bone Joint Surg* 1963;45B:528-541.

4. Rettig AC, Shelbourne KD, McCarroll JR, et al: The natural history and treatment of delayed union stress fractures of the anterior cortex of the tibia. *Am J Sports Med* 1988;16:250-255.
5. Rosen PR, Micheli LJ, Treves S: Early scintigraphic diagnosis of bone stress and fractures in athletic adolescents. *Pediatrics* 1982;70:11-15.
6. Stanitski CL, McMaster JH, Scranton PE: On the nature of stress fractures. *Am J Sports Med* 1978;6:391-396.
7. Yousem D, Magid D, Fishman EK, et al: Computed tomography of stress fractures. *J Comput Assist Tomogr* 1986;10:92-95.
8. Ingersoll CF: Ice skater's fracture. *Radiology* 1943;50:469-479.
9. Jackson DW, Wiltse LL, Cirincione RJ: Spondylolysis in the female gymnast. *Clin Orthop* 1976;117:68-73.
10. Wiltse LL, Widell EH, Jackson DW: Fatigue fracture: The basic lesion in isthmic spondylolisthesis. *J Bone Joint Surg* 1975;57A:17-22.
11. Bruns BR, Yngve DA: Stress reaction and stress fracture, in *Advances in Sports Medicine and Fitness*. Chicago, Yearbook Medical Publishers, vol 2, 1988, pp 201-222.
12. Towne LC, Blazina ME, Cozen LN: Fatigue fracture of the tarsal navicular. *J Bone Joint Surg* 1970;52A:376-378.
13. Mutoh Y, Mori T, Suzuki Y, et al: Stress fractures of the ulna in athletes. *Am J Sports Med* 1982;10:365-367.
14. Rettig AC: Stress fracture of the ulna in an adolescent tournament tennis player. *Am J Sports Med* 1983;11:103-106.
15. Allen ME: Stress fracture of the humerus. *Am J Sports Med* 1974;12:244-245.
16. Dickason JM, Fox JM: Fracture of the patella due to overuse syndrome in a child. *Am J Sports Med* 1982;10:248-249.
17. Matheson GO, Clement DB, McKenzie DC, et al: Stress fractures in athletes. *Am J Sports Med* 1987;15:46-58.
18. Pentecost RL, Murray RA, Brindley HH: Fatigue, insufficiency, and pathologic fractures. *JAMA* 1964;187(13)111-114.
19. Milgrom C, Giladi M, Simkin A, et al: An analysis of the biomechanical mechanism of tibial stress fractures among Israeli infantry recruits. *Clin Orthop* 1988;231:216-221.
20. Rubin CT, Lanyon LE: Osteoregulatory nature of mechanical stimuli: Function as a determinant for adaptive remodeling in bone. *J Orthop Res* 1987;5:300-310.
21. Scully TJ, Besterman G: Stress fracture: A preventable training injury. *Milit Med* 1982;147:285-287.
22. Moritani T, De Vries HA: Neural factors versus hypertrophy in the time course of muscles strength gain. *Am J Phys Med* 1979;58:115-130.
23. Warren MP, Brooks-Gunn J, Hamilton LH, et al: Scoliosis and fractures in young ballet dancers. *New Engl J Med* 1986;314:1348-1353.
24. Troup JDG: Mechanical factors in spondylolisthesis and spondylolysis. *Clin Orthop* 1976;117:59-67.
25. Walsh WM, Huurman WW, Shelton GL: Overuse injuries of the knee and spine in girls' gymnastics. *Orthop Clin North Am* 1985;16:329-350.
26. Roche MB, Rowe GG: The incidence of separate neural arch and coincident bone variations. *J Bone Joint Surg* 1952;34A:491-494.
27. Ferguson RJ: Low-back pain in college football linemen. *J Bone Joint Surg* 1974;56A:1300.
28. Walter NE, Wolf MD: Stress fractures in young athletes. *Am J Sports Med* 1977;5:165-170.

Section Seven

Rehabilitation

Chapter 26

Rehabilitation of the Pediatric Athlete

Kaye E. Wilkins, MD

To determine whether there is a need for extensive rehabilitation programs for pediatric athletes (defined as those whose musculoskeletal growth is incomplete), it is necessary to examine the incidence of sports-related injuries in pediatric athletes, determine if such injuries have any long-lasting physical effects, and identify any changes that have altered the injury rate.

Incidence of Injuries

The Committee on School Health of the American Academy of Pediatrics once thought that body contact sports would increase growth plate injuries and lead to long-term disabilities. In a 1956 policy statement[1] the committee recommended that they be "avoided." Later studies, however, demonstrated that these fears were unfounded. Larson and McMahan[2] found that only 6% of sports-related injuries in children under 14 years old involved the growth plate. Peterson and Peterson[3] showed that the incidence of physeal injuries is age-related. Other studies confirmed that the rate of injury in organized sport activities is low in pediatric athletes but does increase with age. More high-school students than grade-school students are injured.[4-6] Goldberg and associates[5] and Zaricznyj and associates[6] specifically demonstrated that recreational and unsupervised sporting activities were much more likely to produce injuries.

Type of Sport The injury rate is related to the degree of body contact. Football and wrestling cause more injuries than do swimming and tennis.[7,8] Nonetheless, studies of Little League football have shown that fewer than 5% of the reported injuries prevented further participation.[9-11]

Serious central nervous system injuries are rare in children under 15 years old. Head injuries occur in only 230 per 100,000 children per year and spinal cord injuries in only one per 100,000 children per year. However, in adolescents and young adults 15 to 24 years old, there are

349 head injuries per 100,000 participants per year and eight spinal cord injuries per 100,000 participants per year. Automobile accidents and falls are responsible for 60% to 70% of head injuries and almost all spinal injuries in children under 15 years old. Thus, very few children sustain major head or spinal trauma as a result of participating in organized sports.[12]

Bicycles are the primary producers of injuries in children. The injury rate for bicycles and equipment was 812 per 100,000 children, compared with 416 per 100,00 children for football.[13] Another significant cause of deaths and injuries in the primary grades is playground equipment.[14,15]

Long-Lasting Physical Effects

Although many injury patterns can produce long-term effects, in pediatric athletes these are for the most part overuse syndromes rather than traumatic injuries.

In 1965 Adams[16] called attention to the effects of excessive throwing on the immature elbow. Follow-up studies of "Little League elbow," however, later showed that when the rules were changed to decrease the number of pitches, the incidence of long-term disabling injuries was much less.[17-20]

Dominguez[21] noted that almost 50% of the swimmers he examined had shoulder symptoms. Some even had class III, disabling pain.

Roy and associates,[22] in their study of high-performance gymnasts, found that young, growing gymnasts demonstrated distal physeal changes. Those with radiographic changes took at least three months to recover. Those without radiographic changes recovered more quickly (in about four weeks). In neither group, however, were residual growth problems observed.

Mital and associates[23] found that the major long-term effect of Osgood-Schlatter disease (osteochondrosis) is an occasional bony fragment that fails to resolve or unite but responds well to surgical excision.

Except for the reports cited, there have been few long-term studies on the effects of sports injuries in the pediatric athlete.[24]

Factors Decreasing the Incidence of Sports Injuries

Rules and equipment changes have proved to be effective in reducing sports injuries. Guidelines for controlling the number of innings pitched and the types of pitches thrown seem to have decreased the incidence of disability caused by Little League elbow.[17-20] It is hoped that the ban on spearing will decrease the incidence of cervical spine injuries in football.[12] Improvements in football helmets decreased the number of fatal head injuries from 36 in 1968 to nine in 1981.[13]

Another effective way to decrease injuries is to match athletes by size and skill rather than by age.[25]

Rehabilitation Studies

Although recent sports medicine texts contain excellent information on rehabilitation techniques[26-32] and protective equipment,[33,34] less has been published on the specifics of pediatric rehabilitation.[35,36] Some studies have suggested that strength training is beneficial,[37-39] although weight-lifting is considered to be an unsafe sport for children.

Rehabilitation programs have been developed for specific overuse syndromes in pediatric athletes. Kujala and associates[40] discussed knee rehabilitation in Osgood-Schlatter disease and others have studied patellar chondromalacia and Sinding-Larsen disease.[41-43] Metzmaker and Pappas[44] outlined a five-stage program of rehabilitation for apophyseal avulsion injuries around the pelvis. Micheli and Ireland[45] described a program of prevention and rehabilitation of calcaneal apophysitis using orthotics, stretching, and ankle dorsiflexion strengthening. In a review of 14 patients who underwent elbow arthrotomy for osteochondritis of the capitellum, McManama and associates[46] presented a rehabilitation program for the postoperative period.

Rehabilitation Equipment

Although accommodating-resistance and variable-resistance machines are available, they tend to be complicated and expensive, and may be too large for children. Constant-resistance equipment, such as simple weights used in a home gym, are easily adapted for use by children. Because a child's motivation and attention span may present problems, the programs need to be simple and fun.

References

1. American Academy of Pediatrics Committee on School Health: Competitive athletics: A statement of policy. *Pediatrics* 1956;18:672-676.
2. Larson RL, McMahan RO: The epiphyses and the childhood athlete. *JAMA* 1966;196:607-612.
3. Peterson CA, Peterson HA: Analysis of the incidence of injuries to the epiphyseal growth plate. *J Trauma* 1972;12:275-281.
4. Collins HR: Contact sports in junior high school. *Tex Med* 1967;63:67-69.
5. Goldberg B, Witman PA, Gleim GW, et al: Children's sports injuries: Are they avoidable? *Phys Sportsmed* 1979;7:93-101.
6. Zaricznyj B, Shattuck LJ, Mast TA, et al: Sports-related injuries in school-aged children. *Am J Sports Med* 1980;8:318-324.
7. Garrick JG, Requa RK: Injuries in high school sports. *Pediatrics* 1978;61:465-469.
8. Chambers RB: Orthopeadic injuries in athletes (ages 6 to 17): Comparison of injuries occurring in six sports. *Am J Sports Med* 1979;7:195-197.
9. Roser LA, Clawson DK: Football injuries in the very young athlete. *Clin Orthop* 1970;69:219-223.
10. Godshall RW: Junior League football: Risks vs. benefits. *J Sports Med* 1975; 3:139-144.

11. Goldberg B, Rosenthal PP, Nicholas JA: Injuries in youth football. *Phys Sportsmed* 1984;12:122-132.

12. Bruce DA, Schut L, Sutton LN: Brain and cervical spine injuries occurring during organized sports activities in children and adolescents. *Clin Sports Med* 1982;1:495-514.

13. Mueller F, Blyth C: Epidemiology of sports injuries in children. *Clin Sports Med* 1982;1:343-352.

14. Langley JD, Silva PA, Williams SM: Primary school accidents. *NZ Med J* 1981;94:336-339.

15. Nixon J, Pearn J, Wilkey I: Death during play: A study of playground and recreational deaths in children. *Br Med J* 1981;283:410.

16. Adams JE: Injury to the throwing arm: A study of traumatic changes in the elbow joints of boy baseball players. *Calif Med* 1965;102:127-132.

17. Gugenheim JJ Jr, Stanley RF, Woods GW, et al: Little League survey: The Houston study. *Am J Sports Med* 1976;4:189-200.

18. Larson RL, Singer KM, Bergstrom R, et al: Little League survey: The Eugene study. *Am J Sports Med* 1976;4:201-209.

19. Slager RF: From Little League to big league: The weak spot is the arm. *Am J Sports Med* 1977;5:37-48.

20. Francis R, Bunch T, Chandler B: Little League elbow: A decade later. *Phys Sportsmed* 1978;6:88-94.

21. Dominguez RH: Shoulder pain in swimmers. *Phys Sportsmed* 1980;8:35-48.

22. Roy S, Caine D, Singer KM: Stress changes of the distal radial epiphysis in young gymnasts: A report of twenty-one cases and a review of the literature. *Am J Sports Med* 1985;13:301-308.

23. Mital MA, Matza RA, Cohen J: The so-called unresolved Osgood-Schlatter lesion: A concept based on fifteen surgically treated lesions. *J Bone Joint Surg* 1980;62A:732-739.

24. Kozar B, Lord RM: Overuse injury in the young athlete: Reasons for concern. *Phys Sportsmed* 1983;11:116-122.

25. Hafner J: Problems in matching young athletes: Body fat, peach fuzz, muscle and mustache. *Sportsmed* 1985;3:96-98.

26. Kulund DN (ed): *The Injured Athlete*, ed 2. Philadelphia, JP Lippincott, 1988.

27. Appenzeller O (ed): *Sports Medicine: Fitness, Training, Injuries*, ed 3. Baltimore, Urban & Schwarzenberg, 1988.

28. American Academy of Orthopaedic Surgeons: *Athletic Training and Sports Medicine*. Park Ridge, American Academy of Orthopaedic Surgeons, 1984.

29. Perry J: Scientific basis of rehabilitation, in Stauffer ES (ed): American Academy of Orthopaedic Surgeons *Instructional Course Lectures, XXXIV*. St. Louis, CV Mosby, 1985, pp 385-388.

30. Allman FL Jr: Rehabilitative exercises in sports medicine, in Stauffer ES (ed): American Academy of Orthopaedic Surgeons *Instructional Course Lectures, XXXIV*. St. Louis, CV Mosby, 1985, pp 389-392.

31. Grana WA, Karr J, Stafford M: Rehabilitation techniques for athletic injury, in Stauffer ES (ed): American Academy of Orthopaedic Surgeons *Instructional Course Lectures, XXXIV*. St. Louis, CV Mosby, 1985, pp 393-400.

32. Harvey J (ed): *Symposium on Pediatric and Adolescent Sports Medicine*. Philadelphia, WB Saunders, 1982.

33. Vinger PF, Hoerner EF (eds): *Sports Injuries: The Unthwarted Epidemic*. Littleton, Mass, PSG Publishing, 1981.

34. Scott WN, Nisonson B, Nicholas JA (eds): *Principles of Sports Medicine*. Baltimore, Williams & Wilkins, 1984.

35. Martens R, et al (eds): *Coaching Young Athletes*. Champaign, Il, Human Kinetics Publishers, 1981.

36. Micheli LJ (ed): *Injuries in the Young Athlete*. Philadelphia, WB Saunders, 1988.

37. Sewall L, Micheli LJ: Strength training for children. *J Pediatr Orthop* 1986;6:143-146.

38. Duda M: Prepubescent strength training gains support. *Phys Sportsmed* 1986;14:157-161.

39. Rians CB, Weltman A, Cahill BR, et al: Strength training for prepubescent males: Is it safe? *Am J Sports Med* 1987;15:483-489.

40. Kujala UM, Kvist M, Heinonen O: Osgood-Schlatter's disease in adolescent athletes: Retrospective study of incidence and duration. *Am J Sports Med* 1985;13:236-241.

41. James SL: Chondromalacia of the patella in the adolescent, in Kennedy JC (ed): *The Injured Adolescent Knee*. Baltimore, Williams & Wilkins, 1979, ch 8.

42. Larson RL: Subluxation-dislocation of the patella, in Kennedy JC (ed): *The Injured Adolescent Knee*. Baltimore, Williams & Wilkins, 1979, ch 7.

43. Lysholm J, Nordin M, Ekstrand J, et al: The effect of a patella brace on performance in a knee extension strength test in patients with patellar pain. *Am J Sports Med* 1984;12:110-112.

44. Metzmaker JN, Pappas AM: Avulsion fractures of the pelvis. *Am J Sports Med* 1985;13:349-358.

45. Micheli LJ, Ireland ML: Prevention and management of calcaneal apophysitis in children: An overuse syndrome. *J Pediatr Orthop* 1987;7:34-38.

46. McManama GB Jr, Micheli LJ, Berry MV, et al: The surgical treatment of osteochondritis of the capitellum. *Am J Sports Med* 1985;13:11-21.

Chapter 27

A Therapist's View of Rehabilitation in the Pediatric Athlete

Dee Tipton, MPH, PT, ATC

Increased interest in physical fitness and widespread participation in sports have made sports medicine a primary focus for the health-care industry. The possibility of reducing injuries among young athletes has long been the goal of the orthopaedic community. Despite rule changes, improved technology of sports equipment, and better understanding of the mechanics of motion, injuries still occur. What happens to the athlete immediately after injury and subsequent to returning to the activity is of vital importance and can have either positive or negative effects on the child's ability to continue lifelong physical activities.

Injuries occur as a result of a combination of factors including the type of sport, the level of competitive participation, the equipment used, coaching techniques, and playing conditions. These variables interact with the athlete's physical characteristics (size, age, sex, strength, speed, agility, coordination, physical fitness, flexibility, and ligamentous laxity) and personality traits (being conscientious, staid, rule-bound, controlled, tough-minded, reserved, overprotected, or sensitive).[1] Another important consideration is whether the sport is organized or unorganized.[2]

In general, the following steps decrease the frequency and severity of injury: (1) proper and thorough warm-ups and stretching before and after any physical exertion; (2) good conditioning, both preseason and during the season; (3) use of good-quality, well-fitting equipment; (4) good maintenance of playing areas; (5) well-planned, relatively short practices; (6) capable officials; (7) preseason physical examinations; (8) knowledge of first aid by the coach; (9) readiness of the coach to refer the injured child to a physician, and (10) unwillingness to expose any child to undue risk of injury or to aggravation of an existing injury.

Rehabilitation should begin immediately after injury. The control and prevention of hemorrhage, effusion, edema, inflammatory response, and muscle spasm reduce morbidity to the injured area and facilitate an earlier return to full and safe participation.

Importance of Rehabilitation

One of the major contributions the physical therapist or trainer makes to the welfare of the athlete is in rehabilitation. The type of rehabilitation program prescribed may determine the level of athletic participation that is possible in the future.

The most commonly encountered abnormality in the orthopaedic screening evaluation is evidence of inadequate rehabilitation of previous sports injuries. The three most important areas to evaluate are symmetrical muscle development, range of motion, and presence of deformities.[3]

The quality of rehabilitation also influences the frequency of injury. An example comes from a study by the New York Public High School Athletic Association. This study showed that the rate of knee injury was 15 to 17 times greater for those with previously injured knees than for players who had not sustained knee injuries. Most of those reinjured had not had adequate rehabilitation.[4] The West Point study[5] pointed out that 80% of the knee injuries at the Academy occurred in athletes previously injured in high school. Therefore, there is documentation that recognition of a deficiency and its correction or the use of a preventive exercise program will decrease the occurrence of injury in the adolescent or other athlete. Such studies have not been done in the pediatric athlete and there is disagreement about the need for and value of rehabilitation in the pediatric athlete. This is an area in need of further study.

Goals and Objectives of Rehabilitation

The goals in the rehabilitation of an injured athlete are somewhat different from those for the general population. Vigorous, intense, but controlled exercise allows earlier return to activity only if the injured tissues are prepared optimally. According to Allman,[6] the goal of treatment must be to restore function to the greatest possible degree in the shortest possible time.

Rehabilitation begins immediately after injury with early intervention and proper acute care to minimize the physiologic effects of injury. The aim is not to speed up healing, but rather to do everything possible to prevent disuse and deconditioning.[7]

Rehabilitation is influenced by a number of factors.[4] These include the severity of injury, the stage of tissue healing, the type of treatment, the strength of the muscles of the entire limb, pain on motion of the joint, range of joint motion, joint swelling, other conditions within the joint, and the demands that the sport will make on the injured part.

Stages of Rehabilitation

Rehabilitation should proceed in an orderly fashion in a series of steps.[4] Initially, emphasis is on cardiovascular fitness and isometric contractions if the part is immobilized.[8] Exercise of the opposite limb evokes a crossover reaction and maintains the muscles of the opposite limb.[9] If permitted, limited motion within the confines of any restriction helps healing.[10] When any restriction is discontinued, a pain-free range of motion is regained through graded exercise that may include proprioceptive neuromuscular facilitation, transcutaneous electrical stimulation, and cold applications. Each of these techniques is used to overcome the neural inhibition that limits progress at this stage.[11] As joint motion and flexibility return, resistance exercise is increased by using light weights and many repetitions done at less than maximal effort. As strength is developed, more emphasis is placed on speed, power, endurance, and flexibility. Finally, specific skill patterns and sport-related skills are prescribed.

Criteria for Return to Activity

Several criteria should be monitored during and at the end of the rehabilitation program. These criteria are generally based on measurements of the uninvolved side. They include the strength, power, and endurance of each muscle group; the balance between antagonistic muscle groups, such as the quadriceps-hamstring ratio in the thigh muscles; the flexibility of the soft tissue around the rehabilitated joint and any restriction contracture; and, finally, the return of proprioception of the injured joint and limb by progressive functional activity until the skills required in the sport are attained.

Common Mistakes in Rehabilitation

Five mistakes are common during rehabilitation, but all can be avoided with proper supervision. (1) Rehabilitation is often focused on a single muscle group rather than offering an integrated approach that includes antagonistic muscle groups of the entire limb. (2) Rehabilitation is often discontinued before the injured limb's performance is equal to or better than that of the uninjured side. (3) Exercises to develop proprioception are often forgotten and, therefore, the key link to function is neglected. (4) Postural defects and anatomic malalignment, as well as biomechanical imbalances, are frequently neglected as the rehabilitation program is developed. (5) Sport-specific skills and the SAID principle (specific adaptation to imposed demands) are not incorporated into the program. Exercise should be adapted to the specific needs of the athlete's particular position and/or sport.[5]

Summary

Despite the best efforts of athletes, coaches, parents, and therapists, injuries do occur. Rehabilitation, therefore, is needed to return the athlete to his or her sport. Supervised rehabilitation has a role in the treatment of the pediatric athlete. Exactly what that role is remains a matter of judgment because no scientific information documenting the best type, amount, and duration of the rehabilitation program is available.

References

1. Jackson D, Jarrett H, Bailey D: *Am J Sports Med* 1978;6:6-14.
2. Zaricznyj B, Shattock L: *Am J Sports Med* 1980;8:318-324.
3. Smith N: Chicago, Year Book Medical Publishers, 1981, pp 187-227.
4. Roy S, Irwin R: *Sports Medicine*. Englewood Cliffs, Calif, Prentice-Hall, 1983.
5. Abbott HG, Kress JB: Preconditioning in the conditioning of knee injuries. *Arch Phys Med Rehab* 1969;50:326-333.
6. Allman FL in Ryan AJ, Allman FL (eds): *Sports Medicine*. New York, Academic Press, 1974.
7. Leach RE: The prevention and rehabilitation of soft tissue injuries. *Int Sports Med* 1982;3:18-20.
8. Heltinger ERT, Muller EA: Influence of training and of inactivity on muscle strength. *Arch Phys Med* 1962;41:45-55.
9. Hellebrandt FA, Waterland JC: Indirect learning: The influence of unimanual exercise on related muscle groups of the same and the opposite side. *Am J Phys Med* 1962;41:45-55.
10. Tipton CM, Matthes RO, Maynard JA, et al: The influence of physical activity on ligaments and tendons. *Med Sci Sports* 1975;7:165-175.
11. Aten DW, Knight KL: Therapeutic exercise in athletic training: Principles and overview. *Ath Train* 1978;13:112-126.

Consensus Statements: Rehabilitation

1. The incidence of disabling injuries in the skeletally immature athlete (elementary and junior high) is low.
2. Given the above, there is less need for extensive rehabilitation programs for this age group.
3. Failure to rehabilitate the athlete fully prior to re-entry can contribute to re-injury.
4. Overuse syndromes cause many of the problems that affect the skeletally immature athlete.
    (a). Emphasis on prevention and treatment of the overuse syndromes is needed.
    (b). Research is needed on the long-term effects of overuse and other pediatric injuries.
5. There is scant research or literature on rehabilitation of the pediatric athlete or on equipment specifically designed for rehabilitation in this age group. Support of such research must be encouraged.

Section Eight

Protective Equipment

Chapter 28

Protective Equipment

Kaye E. Wilkins, MD

Any discussion of protective equipment must evaluate the effects of using such equipment, consider the role of certifying agencies, and attempt to provide principles of selection.

Equipment

Football

Helmets   Football helmets have evolved from the leather helmets with internal suspension used in the 1930s and the rigid outer shells with webbed suspension used in the 1950s.[1] Modern helmets consist of rigid outer shells with padded pneumatic and hydraulic systems.

There is documented evidence of decreased direct fatalities, head injuries associated with cranial hemorrhage, and injuries associated with death over the past two decades. Torg and associates[2] attribute this to the increased effectiveness of the helmet/face-mask system. This very effectiveness, however, has led to an increase in cervical spine fractures and dislocations that result in permanent quadriplegia. Protecting the head allows it to be used as a battering ram, thus placing the cervical spine at risk.[2] The hardness of the helmets has contributed to more injuries from direct blows, including fractures of the extremities and ribs and facial injuries.[3] Padding the helmet with a soft covering might decrease the incidence of this direct trauma.

The increased bulkiness of the newer suspension systems diminishes the area available for heat loss. Because of this heat retention, players should remove their helmets when they are on the sidelines.[4]

Cineradiographic studies have shown that the helmet does not affect the cervical spine directly. Rather, the hyperflexion of the spine indirectly causes cervical fracture-dislocations.[5] Andrish and associates[6] showed that the addition of a simple flexion strap attached to the shoulder pads can decrease flexion movements. This strap seemed to be especially effective in preventing recurrence of injuries in patients who had previous neck injuries.

Although face masks have decreased the number of facial injuries, they can also cause injuries.[7] Current models have a double or single bar for backfield players, whereas those who play on the line wear a cage style.[8] A bar placed too low exposes the face, and one placed too high obstructs vision. A bar too close to the face can be driven back into the face during violent contact. The face mask should be connected to the helmet by rubber attachments that help absorb shock and allow easy removal in emergencies.

Chin straps should have four-point fixation to prevent helmet rotation[1] and should also prevent lateral rotation.

Mouth Guards   Mouth and other facial injuries once accounted for 50% of all football injuries. Face guards have cut the number of injuries in half. With the added use of mouth guards, the incidence of dental injuries is now less than 1%.[9]

There is also good evidence to show that custom-fabricated protectors decrease the intracranial pressure generated by a direct blow to the jaw.[10]

Mouth guards are of three basic types: (1) Stock guards are made of materials other than thermoplastic. They are inexpensive but do not fit well and players often fail to wear them. (2) Mouth-formed guards are made of resin that softens in hot water and adapts to the mouth. This type is very bulky and often uncomfortable. (3) Custom-made guards are the most expensive. Because they are made by dentists or dental technicians from an impression of the maxillary arch, they are the most comfortable type and have the best compliance rate.[9,11] The best material for fabrication appears to be a laminated thermoplastic material. This was found to be superior to the more commonly used polycopolymers.[12]

Mouth guards are often not worn because they fit poorly and are uncomfortable. Additionally, the players may be poorly educated about their importance. An effective mouth guard must be fitted properly, used only by the player it belongs to, not interfere with speech, and be securely attached to the helmet.[12]

Mouth guards are also recommended for other sports such as ice hockey, basketball, field hockey, lacrosse, wrestling, skiing, baseball, rugby, and soccer.

Shoes   Hightop shoes decrease the load placed on the collateral ligaments.[13] If shoes other than hightops are used for mobility, the subtalar joint must be free to move. This lessens the strain on the collateral ligaments. Garrick and Requa[14] found that the combination of hightop shoes and taping decreased the incidence of recurrent ankle sprains without increasing the incidence of knee injuries.

Studies by Torg and associates[15] demonstrated that the safest football shoe for all surfaces has a rigid synthetic sole molded with 15 cleats, each 0.5 inch in length, and a tip 0.5 inch in diameter. Mueller and Blythe[16] found that short and long cleats produced similar injury rates in poorly maintained fields but that the shorter cleats apparently decreased the incidence of injuries in fields that were in good condition. They believe that both good shoes and well-maintained fields are needed to prevent ankle and knee injuries.

Other Sports Equipment

Shin Guards   Shin guards protect against tibial fractures caused by direct blows, one of the most common soccer injuries.[17,18] Shin guards will be required worldwide by the governing body of soccer after the 1990 World Cup.

Baseball Equipment   Baseball helmets decrease the incidence of head injuries. Throat guards for catchers decrease the incidence of neck injuries. Breakaway bases and the prohibition against sliding in Little League games have decreased the incidence of ankle injuries.[19]

Protective Eye Equipment   Such equipment should be used by anyone playing squash, racketball, or handball.[20]

Bicycle Helmets   Head injuries constitute the greatest cause of death and injury in bicycle accidents. Unfortunately, there are no controlled studies demonstrating that a bicycle helmet protects against head injury. Although it has been recommended that helmets be worn when riding bicycles,[21] very young children may not understand the need for bicycle helmets.[22]

Equipment That Is Not Helpful

Knee Braces   Studies have shown that knee braces do not protect the knee effectively.[23,24] In addition, there is an increased incidence of ankle injuries in players using knee braces.[23,24]

Artificial Turf   This new surface has increased the incidence of skin burns, contusions, strains, and traumatic bursitis.[25-28]

Fiberglass Poles   The new fiberglass poles used in pole vaulting, along with improvements in runways and planting techniques, have increased performance so much that landing surfaces now require more shock-absorbing qualities.[29]

Certifying and Testing Organizations

Considerable research has been devoted to establishing the minimum standards necessary to produce effective but reasonably priced equipment.[29,30] Providing total safety would impair performance in many cases to an unacceptable level. Thus, compromises may be necessary in establishing standards. Recently, medicolegal concerns have become a major factor in the production of athletic equipment.

The Consumer Products Safety Commission (CPSC) is the major government agency dealing with the safety of consumer products. This agency provides the National Electronic Injury Surveillance System (NEISS), which collects data on product-related injuries from hospital emergency rooms. This reporting system shows that use of bicycle- and football-related equipment during these activities produces the highest injury rates.

The American Society for Testing Materials (ASTM) is a large organization founded in 1898 to develop voluntary standards for various consumer products. It includes manufacturers, consumers, academicians, medical authorities, and government representatives. In 1969 a committee on sports equipment facilities was established to produce standards for athletic equipment. This committee has 15 subcommittees that specialize in areas such as football, hockey, playing surfaces, headwear, and footwear. Products manufactured to ASTM standards have already met some safety requirements.

The National Operating Committee on Standards for Athletic Equipment (NOCSAE) was established in 1969 to develop safety standards for athletic equipment. It initially established standards for football helmets for the National Collegiate Athletic Association and the National Federation of State High School Associations. This group placed a warning label on helmets and is now studying baseball helmets and football face guards.

The National Athletic Equipment Reconditioners Association (NAERA) tests used equipment to be sure that the National Operating Committee's standards are met.

The effectiveness of these certification agencies is shown by the fact that since the Hockey Equipment Certification Council set standards for hockey face masks and mandated the use of certified equipment, no injuries have led to loss of sight.

Principles of Selection

Safety should be the first consideration in selecting sports equipment; cost and appearance are less important. Secondhand equipment should not be used unless it has been recertified. All equipment should be manufactured by a reputable company and certified by one of the accepted agencies. Equipment should not improve performance at the expense of safety. Equipment should fit properly, and coaches, trainers, players, and physicians all need to be trained in its proper use. The kind of equipment used may have to change in response to technological advances.[29]

References

1. Park J, Arnold JA: Protective athletic equipment. *J Ark Med Soc* 1977;74:202-204.
2. Torg JS, Truex R Jr, Quedenfeld TC, et al: The National Football Head and Neck Injury Registry: Report and conclusions, 1978. *JAMA* 1979;241:1477-1479.
3. Robey JM: Contribution of design and construction of football helmets to the occurrence of injuries. *Med Sci Sports* 1972;4:170-174.
4. Coleman AE, Mortagy AK: Ambient head temperature and football helmet design. *Med Sci Sports* 1973;5:204-208.
5. Virgin H: Cineradiographic study of football helmets and the cervical spine. *Am J Sports Med* 1980;8:310-317.
6. Andrish JT, Bergfeld JA, Romo LR: A method for the management of cervical injuries in football: A preliminary report. *Am J Sports Med* 1977;5:89-92.
7. Wilson K, Rontal E, Rontal M: Facial injuries in football. *Trans Am Acad Ophthalmol Otolaryngol* 1973;77:434-437.

8. Gieck J, McCue FC III: Fitting of protective football equipment. *Am J Sports Med* 1980;8:192-196.

9. Bureau of Dental Health Education, Council on Dental Materials and Devices: Mouth protectors: 11 years later. *JADA* 1973;86:1365-1367.

10. Hickey JC, Morris AL, Carlson LD, et al: The relation of mouth protectors to cranial pressure and deformation. *JADA* 1967;74:735-740.

11. Upson N: Mouthguards: An evaluation of two types for rugby players. *Br J Sports Med* 1985;19:89-92.

12. Chaconas SJ, Caputo AA, Bakke NK: A comparison of athletic mouthguard materials. *Am J Sports Med* 1985;13:193-197.

13. Johnson GR, Dowson D, Wright V: Ankle loading and football boots. *Rheumatol Rehabil* 1976;15:194-196.

14. Garrick JG, Requa RK: Role of external support in the prevention of ankle sprains. *Med Sci Sports* 1973;5:200-203.

15. Torg JS, Quedenfeld TC, Landau S: The shoe-surface interface and its relationship to football knee injuries. *Am J Sports Med* 1974;2:261-269.

16. Mueller FO, Blyth CS: North Carolina high school football injury study: Equipment and prevention. *J Sports Med* 1974;2:1-10.

17. Sullivan JA, Gross RH, Grana WA, et al: Evaluation of injuries in youth soccer. *Am J Sports Med* 1980;8:325-327.

18. Nilsson S, Roaas A: Soccer injuries in adolescents. *Am J Sports Med* 1978;6:358-361.

19. Hale CJ: Protective equipment for baseball. *Phys Sportsmed* 1979;7:59-63.

20. Diamond GR, Quinn GE, Pashby TJ, et al: Ophthalmologic injuries. *Clin Sports Med* 1982;1:469-482.

21. Friede AM, Azzara CV, Gallagher SS, et al: The epidemiology of injuries to bicycle riders. *Pediatr Clin North Am* 1985;32:141-151.

22. Weiss BD: Bicycle helmet use by children. *Pediatrics* 1986;77:677-679.

23. Grace TG, Skipper BJ, Newberry JC, et al: Prophylactic knee braces and injury to the lower extremity. *J Bone Joint Surg* 1988;70A:422-427.

24. Garrick JG, Requa RK: Prophylactic knee bracing. *Am J Sports Med* 1987;15:471-476.

25. Hirata I: *The Doctor and the Athlete*, ed 2. Philadelphia, JB Lippincott, 1974.

26. Bonstingl RW, Morehouse CA, Niebel BW: Torques developed by different types of shoes on various playing surfaces. *Med Sci Sports* 1975;7:127-131.

27. Bowers KD Jr, Martin RB: Turf-toe: A shoe-surface related football injury. *Med Sci Sports* 1976;8:81-83.

28. Larson RL, Osternig LR: Traumatic bursitis and artificial turf. *J Sports Med* 1974;2:183-188.

29. Rosenthal PR: Sports equipment standards, in Scott WN, Nisonson B, Nicholas JA (eds): *Principles of Sports Medicine*. Baltimore, Williams & Wilkins, 1984.

30. Vinger PF, Hoerner EF (eds): *Sports Injuries: The Unthwarted Epidemic*, ed 2. Littleton, Mass, PSG Publishing Co, 1986.

Consensus Statements: Protective Equipment

1. Protective equipment, when used properly, decreases the incidence of injuries.
2. Most athletes, coaches, parents, and support personnel (including team doctors) probably do not fully understand the basic principles involved in the use of protective equipment.
3. Education programs are needed to improve the proper understanding and use of protective equipment.
4. Education programs are also needed to alert the public regarding the value of protective equipment in nonorganized recreational pursuits such as bicycling and skateboarding.
5. The value of certifying agencies should be acknowledged, and only certified equipment should be used.
6. The cost of medicolegal aspects of protective equipment use must be evaluated.
7. Research is necessary to validate the need for protective equipment currently in use, as well as for proposed changes in equipment use (e.g., Do knee braces prevent injuries?).

Index